T0292597

Fundoplication Surgery

Ralph W. Aye • John G. Hunter

Editors

Fundoplication Surgery

A Clinical Guide to Optimizing Results

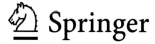 Springer

Editors
Ralph W. Aye, M.D., F.A.C.S.
Staff Thoracic and Esophageal Surgeon
Clinical Program Leader, Thoracic
  Oncology
Fellowship Director, Minimally Invasive
  Thoracic and Esophageal Surgery
Chair, Quality Committee, Swedish Cancer
  Institute
Swedish Medical Center and Swedish
  Cancer Institute
Thoracic and Foregut Surgery
Seattle, WA, USA

John G. Hunter, M.D., F.A.C.S., F.R.C.S.
  Edin (Hon)
Mackenzie Professsor and Chair, Surgery
Editor in Chief, World Journal of Surgery
Oregon Health and Science University
Portland, OR, USA

ISBN 978-3-319-25092-2   ISBN 978-3-319-25094-6   (eBook)
DOI 10.1007/978-3-319-25094-6

Library of Congress Control Number: 2015958806

Springer Cham Heidelberg New York Dordrecht London

Springer International Publishing AG Switzerland is part of Springer Science+Business Media (www.springer.com)

Preface

If you are exploring this book, you are likely aware that gastroesophageal reflux is the most common disorder of the upper intestinal track, and that its impact on our health care system is tremendous, resulting in billions of dollars of medical expenses and lost productivity annually. You may also be vaguely aware, or personally so through the care of your own patients, that antireflux surgery may have a dramatic positive impact on an individual's quality of life, but that, curiously, it has not been fully embraced by the medical community or the public. In fact, medical literature and public online forums are replete with reports of postoperative resumption of antisecretory medication, failed repairs, and debilitating side effects.

As one who has practiced in this arena of surgical endeavor for over 25 years, I find it to be one of the most enjoyable aspects of my practice, because of the substantial and long-lasting improvement in quality of life that I see in the vast majority of patients, and I know that that experience is shared by a great many esophageal surgeons. At the same time, we must acknowledge that the surgical community has sometimes failed in its mission of treating a chronic debilitating benign disease, by limiting our responsibility to the performance of a simple one-size-fits-all operation, with little thought to the subtleties of patient selection, preoperative evaluation, long-term postoperative support and management, and the considerable complexities of the anatomy and physiology of the antireflux barrier and its implications for the creation of a successful repair which will last a patient's lifetime.

This book is an effort to address some of those deficiencies. It is intended for surgeons already performing antireflux procedures who want to elevate their skills to the expert level or for those in their training who want to go beyond the basics. The topics have been selected to address the entire spectrum of the management of gastroesophageal reflux disease, as it is our belief that surgeons who aspire to excellence in this field should understand the complete disease process and its comprehensive management. In addition, the authors have been asked to go beyond the usual textbook descriptions, to share their secrets, their "pearls," and their wisdom from their years of experience in achieving consistently good results and in building the trust of their medical colleagues.

Drs. Schneider and Louie's chapter on the anatomy and physiology of the antireflux barrier is a strongly referenced and in-depth articulation of the current state of our understanding, going far beyond typical references to lower esophageal sphincter pressure and the intra-abdominal esophagus to include detailed anatomy of the complex structure of the LES; the oft-overlooked gastroesophageal valve; the phrenoesophageal membrane, e.g., the substrate holding it all together; and the previously unrecognized substantial importance of the diaphragmatic hiatus as a component of the lower esophageal high pressure zone. An understanding of what it is that we are attempting to reconstruct with our operations is foundational to achieving consistently good outcomes in the face of tremendous anatomic variation.

The centrality of Dr. Hunter and company's chapter on patient selection is hard to overemphasize. A well-performed operation on the wrong patient is a recipe for disaster. The surgeon should understand the complex nuances of an insightful history, the subtexts behind the results of diagnostic studies, and how to apply it all in a specific patient who reflects the substantial variation of individuality. The chapter is masterful and comprehensive, pointing out that there is no shortcut to the diligence and skill required to choose patients appropriately. It should be read more than once to fully appreciate the depth of information packed into its well-written phrasing.

A number of technique-oriented chapters follow. While the interpretation of the concept of short esophagus and its management remains diverse, there is no doubt that cephalad or axial tension on a fundoplication is one of its greatest enemies. Dr. DeMeester et al. have given a state-of-the-art description of its definition and identification, as well as a very well-formed management strategy with which any surgeon performing all but the most straightforward cases should be fully versed, as there is no study which can fully predict in advance whether a shortened esophagus will be encountered. The chapter by Dr. Oelschlager/Wright et al. on difficult diaphragmatic closure expertly addresses a challenging issue which surgeons continue to grapple with. Their discussion of this issue and the options for management come from one of the most well-informed centers in the world on this issue.

Dr. Soper has given a masterful chapter on the proper performance of a Nissen fundoplication. Not only are the specific stepwise details of the operation well articulated and clear, but he has also shared his personal "pitfalls and pearls," gained from the performance of thousands of repairs over many years. While there are many variations in the performance of a Nissen fundoplication, this chapter should remain a reference for all surgeons engaged in antireflux surgery.

Next follow several alternatives to the Nissen wrap. While the Nissen procedure has been to a large extent the international gold standard, it is an aggressive 360° wrap which is typically associated with difficulty belching or vomiting, and this often results in flatulence and to some extent bloating. And despite its aggressiveness, recurrences occur in the best of hands, at a rate higher than we would like to admit. It is because of these issues that several alternatives to the Nissen have been included. My long and fruitful association with Dr. Hill led to an in-depth understanding of his operation and the anatomic components underlying it, and an analysis of failure patterns from our randomized trial comparing the Hill and the Nissen resulted in the development of the Nissen–Hill hybrid repair, in an effort to gain from the strengths of the two individual operations.

Other parts of the world have enjoyed greater success with the Toupet repair than is generally reported in North America, where it is more often used as a compromise procedure in a patient with poor motility. However, Dr. Gotley has explored the pros and cons of both the Nissen and the Toupet in depth and now favors the Toupet as his operation of choice. His detailed description of the procedure is excellent, he has shared his wisdom from a vast experience, and he has honestly reported his results as well as culling a number of comparative studies from the literature. I thoroughly enjoyed his chapter.

While in North America our emphasis as a hallmark of the success of an operation has tended toward control of reflux and the results of postoperative pH measurements, Dr. Watson addresses the vital importance of considering the whole patient, including a recognition of the detrimental impact of fundoplication side effects on patient satisfaction. His pioneering operation, including the results of a number of his own randomized trials, together with a careful reporting of outcomes, is impressive, particularly with regard to global measures of patient satisfaction. In addition, the details of his operation are sufficiently different from standard Nissen technique that one's tool chest for the management of difficult complex situations is expanded.

Dr. Swanstrom's chapter on postoperative management and follow-up is more than I had hoped for with regard to his generous sharing of wisdom, perspective, and specific practical advice in managing the issues that frequently arise after the incisions are closed. This is a critical component of patient management which should not be relegated to the referring physician. In addition, he rightly challenges us all to build reproducible standardized metrics into our practice of a field which is inherently subjective and individualistic. My own experience fully endorses the approach he describes.

Dr. Spechler has been sufficiently kind and direct in his contribution to this book in giving surgeons the perspective of a highly knowledgeable gastroenterologist, helping us to see gastroesophageal reflux disease through the eyes of his colleagues. His central message is clear: it's not just about performing an operation. The majority of patients with reflux do quite well with medical management, and unless the surgeon understands the proper role of antireflux surgery within the broad spectrum of the disease, the elective nature of surgery as an alternative to long-term medical management, and the critical components of patient selection, as well as owning the consequences of the operation, he or she will find it difficult to gain credibility with referring physicians.

Finally, Dr. Jackson helps us to understand the disease process from a pediatric perspective. The importance of this is severalfold. Some of us care for pediatric patients in our practices; this chapter will be invaluable. Secondly it is not uncommon for our adult patients with reflux to describe onset in childhood or teen years. But most excitingly, pediatric surgeons may be ahead of the rest of us in their understanding of the critical role of the phrenoesophageal membrane in maintaining the antireflux barrier. Given the patterns of recurrences we see in our adult patients, regardless of the initial size of the hernia, we may need to pay more attention to this component of our repair. This is alluded to in Dr. Gotley's chapter as well.

As this book has been written with the serious surgeon in mind, "pearls" in most chapters have been emphasized in italics to help identify the author's critical points. Some chapters did not lend themselves to this approach, and for others, like those of Dr. Swanstrom or Dr. Spechler, the entire chapter is a pearl and it was hard to limit emphasis to a few points.

Those of us who have seen firsthand the remarkably beneficial impact of antireflux surgery on well-selected patients know how important it is to get the message across to our medical colleagues and the public. This book is an effort to help you to do so. The authors hope that the information will be of direct value to you in your practice and will result in a benefit to many patients.

Seattle, WA   Ralph W. Aye
Portland, OR   John G. Hunter

Contents

Contributors

Ralph W. Aye, M.D., F.A.C.S. Department of Thoracic and Foregut Surgery, Swedish Cancer Institute, Swedish Medical Center, Seattle, WA, USA

Joshua A. Boys, M.D. Department of Surgery, University of Southern California, Los Angeles, CA, USA

Steven R. DeMeester, M.D. Department of Surgery, University of Southern California, Los Angeles, CA, USA

David Gotley, M.B.B.S., M.D., F.R.A.C.S. Princess Alexandra and Mater Private Hospitals, University of Queensland, Brisbane, QLD, Australia

Department of Surgery, Princess Alexandra Hospital, University of Queensland, Brisbane, QLD, Australia

Kelly R. Haisley, M.D. Department of Surgery, Oregon Health and Science University, Portland, OR, USA

John G. Hunter, M.D. Department of Surgery, Oregon Health and Science University, Portland, OR, USA

Gretchen Purcell Jackson, M.D., Ph.D. Department of Pediatric Surgery, Monroe Carell Jr. Children's Hospital at Vanderbilt, Nashville, TN, USA

Brian E. Louie, M.D., M.H.A., M.P.H., F.R.C.S.C., F.A.C.S. Division of Thoracic Surgery, Swedish Cancer Institute, Swedish Medical Center, Seattle, WA, USA

Brant Oelschlager, M.D. Department of Surgery, University of Washington, Seattle, WA, USA

Andreas M. Schneider, M.D. Division of Thoracic Surgery, Swedish Cancer Institute, Swedish Medical Center, Seattle, WA, USA

Nathaniel J. Soper, M.D. Department of Surgery, Northwestern Memorial Hospital, Chicago, IL, USA

Stuart Jon Spechler, M.D. Department of Medicine, Esophageal Diseases Center, VA North Texas Healthcare System, University of Texas Southwestern Medical Center, Dallas, TX, USA

Division of Gastroenterology and Hepatology (111B1), Dallas VA Medical Center, Dallas, TX, USA

Lee L. Swanstrom, M.D., F.A.C.S., F.A.S.G.E. Institut Hospitalo Universitaire— Strasbourg, 1, place de l'Hopital, Strasbourg, France

Division of GI/MIS, The Oregon Clinic—Gastrointestinal & Minimally Invasive Surgery, Portland, OR, USA

Sergio A. Toledo-Valdovinos, M.D. Department of Surgery, Oregon Health and Science University, Portland, OR, USA

Björn Törnqvist, M.D., Ph.D. Department of Upper Gastrointestinal Surgery, Karolinska University Hospital, Stockholm, Sweden

Heather Warren, M.D. Department of Thoracic Surgery, Swedish Medical Center, Seattle, WA, USA

David I. Watson, M.B.B.S., M.D., F.R.A.C.S., F.A.H.M.S. Flinders University Department of Surgery, Flinders Medical Centre, Adelaide, South Australia, Australia

Stephanie G. Worrell, M.D. Division of Thoracic Surgery, Department of Surgery, Keck School of Medicine of the University of Southern California, Los Angeles, CA, USA

Andrew Wright, M.D. Department of Surgery, University of Washington, Seattle, WA, USA

Robert B. Yates, M.D. Department of Surgery, University of Washington, Seattle, WA, USA

Chapter 1
Anatomy of the Reflux Barrier in Health, Disease, and Reconstruction

Andreas M. Schneider and Brian E. Louie

Introduction

The junction between the esophagus and the stomach is one of the most dynamic areas in the human body. At this junction, ingested food and liquids must be allowed to easily pass into the stomach to initiate the digestive process. At the same time, it must prevent retrograde passage of gastric contents into the esophagus over a wide variety of bodily positions and pressure changes. This simple concept works well for the majority of people with infrequent and often minor disruptions, but a dysfunctional and defective reflux barrier can lead to significant symptoms of gastroesophageal reflux. This disease plagues 18.1–59 % of the US population at least weekly [1, 2], consumes over $7.7 billion in drug costs annually [3], and results in lost productivity, estimated at over $14.6 billion annually [4]. In this chapter, we will examine the components of the reflux barrier in health and disease, discuss the pathophysiology leading to deterioration of the reflux barrier and thus GERD, and highlight potential pitfalls of the reconstructed reflux barrier that are discussed in subsequent chapters.

The Elusive Lower Esophageal Sphincter

Prior to the 1950s, there was considerable controversy surrounding the presence or absence of a lower esophageal sphincter (LES). The earliest description supporting the presence of a sphincter is credited to Helviticus in the 1700s, although not much is known about this description. Despite an intuitive understanding of a valve

A.M. Schneider, M.D. • B.E. Louie, MD, MHA, MPH, FRCSC, FACS (✉)
Division of Thoracic Surgery, Swedish Cancer Institute, Swedish Medical Center,
1101 Madison Street, Suite 900, Seattle, WA 98105, USA
e-mail: andreas.schneider@swedish.org; brian.louie@swedish.org

© Springer International Publishing Switzerland 2016   1
R.W. Aye, J.G. Hunter (eds.), *Fundoplication Surgery*,
DOI 10.1007/978-3-319-25094-6_1

function that prevented reflux of gastric contents, it remained difficult to identify a clear anatomic structure in humans that corresponded to a physiological sphincter. With the advancement of radiology and increasing use of barium, an extensive investigation of the LES began with varying results. Different theories argued for or against the existence of a LES. Some authors felt that the diaphragm acted as the reflux barrier by forming a pinchcock valve on the esophagus [5]. An actively contracting mucosal membrane was suspected to add to the barrier by some [6], whereas others regarded the esophageal contractions seen on barium swallow as a reflexive reaction to distension [7]. These arguments debating the presence or absence of a physiologic sphincter mechanism lasted until the 1950s.

Evidence of a Sphincter

Physiological evidence of a sphincter improved with the development of a pressure catheter similar to modern manometry. This allowed the identification of a high pressure zone within 2–3 cm of the gastroesophageal junction [8]. Using the pressure catheter concomitantly with radiographic images, the "high-pressure" zone was localized approximately 0.5–1 cm above and below the diaphragmatic hiatus. The pressure in this area remained very constant even when the patient's intra-abdominal pressure increased or they were placed in a head-down position [9]. The only time a pressure decrease occurred was with deglutition. These initial findings laid down the fundamental knowledge in our understanding of what is now known today as the LES.

Despite this, skepticism about its anatomical correlation persisted. Ex vivo, the otherwise tonic LES was not palpable, and on pathological examination, its delicate muscle fibers retracted upon transection making their identification and potential orientation very difficult on histological review. There had been prior descriptions of thickening of the circular muscle layers [10], but only when specimens of the distal esophagus and stomach were fixated and micro-dissected [11] were the extensions of the muscularis propria that realigned themselves at the gastroesophageal junction to form the so-called clasp and semi-oblique sling fibers clearly identified. These horizontal C-shaped clasp fibers and the semi-oblique sling fibers form an asymmetrical sphincter, and its functional correlation with the manometric high pressure zone has been proven with different studies (Fig. 1.1) [12, 13].

Components of the Reflux Barrier

In the modern era, there are four main components that function together to form the reflux barrier: the LES, especially its overall and intra-abdominal length; the flap valve enforced by the angle of His; the crural diaphragm or hiatal canal; and the phrenoesophageal ligament (Fig. 1.2).

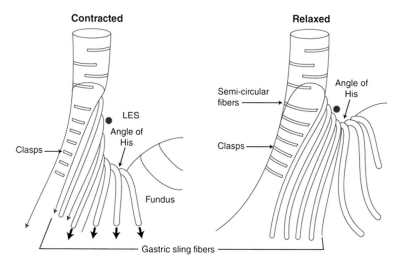

Fig. 1.1 Function of the clasp and sling fibers. *Source*: Surgical Endoscopy April 2015, Volume 29, Issue 4, pp 796–804, 24 Jul 2014, Assessment and reduction of diaphragmatic tension during hiatal hernia repair, © Springer Science+Business Media New York 2014, Daniel Davila Bradley, Brian E. Louie, Alexander S. Farivar, Candice L. Wilshire, Peter U. Baik, Ralph W. Aye, Fig. 1 page 797, With permission of Springer Science+Business Media

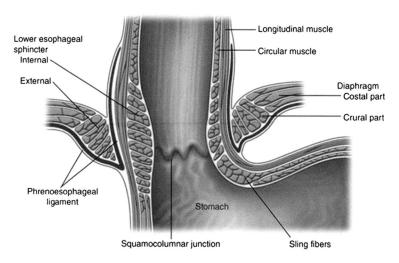

Fig. 1.2 Anatomy of the reflux barrier. *Source*: Surgical Endoscopy April 2015, Volume 29, Issue 4, pp 796–804, 24 Jul 2014, Assessment and reduction of diaphragmatic tension during hiatal hernia repair, © Springer Science+Business Media New York 2014, Daniel Davila Bradley, Brian E. Louie, Alexander S. Farivar, Candice L. Wilshire, Peter U. Baik, Ralph W. Aye, Fig. 3 page 798, With permission of Springer Science+Business Media

LES Length and Pressure

The most studied component of the reflux barrier is the 2–3 cm high pressure zone or LES because it lends itself to an easy pressure measurement. The competence of the barrier is due to a dynamic relationship between the overall length, intra-abdominal length, and the resultant LES pressure (Fig. 1.3) [14]. But, it is important to note at the outset that the pressures observed with manometry likely reflect the contributions of the other components of the reflux barrier described below particularly in the normal state.

This understanding is a result of a series of studies combining pH testing and manometry and was completed in patients with and without symptoms of GERD. First, patients without GERD symptoms or hiatal hernia were compared to patients with GERD/no hernia; GERD with hiatal hernia and after Nissen fundoplication using manometry. Normal patients were found to have a longer sphincter length, approximately 60 % of which was intra-abdominal, and a higher pressure in the LES region, whereas patients with GERD/no hernia had shorter lengths and lower pressures, and those with a hiatal hernia had the shortest length and lowest pressure. Second, when pH studies looking at distal esophageal acid exposures were added to the evaluation, it revealed that with a smaller proportion of esophagus contained in the abdomen, there were higher levels of acid found in the distal esophagus. In addition, acid exposure was inversely proportional to the pressure applied by the LES [15, 16]. Third, the distal esophageal sphincter pressure to intra-gastric pressure ratio required to maintain competency is inversely related to sphincter length (Fig. 1.4) [16].

In summary, over 75 % of subjects with LES pressures less than 6 mmHg had abnormal pH studies, with similar results for abdominal LES length less than 1 cm and overall LES length less than 2 cm. This was used as the physiological basis for developing and refining many of the modern antireflux procedures, especially the Nissen fundoplication.

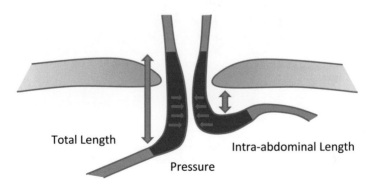

Fig. 1.3 Determinants of competency

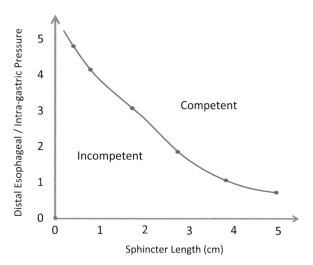

Fig. 1.4 Correlation between pressure and sphincter length. With permission: Elsevier, Inc, Southwestern Surgical Congress, et al. Bonavina L, Evander A, DeMeester TR, Walther B, Cheng S, Palazzo L, et al. Length of the Distal Esophageal Sphincter and Competency of the Cardia. Am J Surg. 1986;151:25–34. Vol 151, January 1986, Fig. 4

Angle of His

Since the extent of intra-abdominal—and related intragastric—pressure generated by valsalva or straining is considerably higher than normal LES pressures, there clearly are other components at work in maintaining competence of the reflux barrier. The angle of esophageal insertion, or angle of His, into the stomach plays a role in maintaining an effective reflux barrier by creating a functional flap valve. This concept was popular and under study at the end of the nineteenth century [17–19]. This concept was revised by Thor and Hill in 1987 in a series of cadaver experiments. They showed that accentuation of the valve via a gastroplasty can increase the pressure in the ex vivo non-tonic LES [20]. Similarly, reduction of the angle through downward fundic pressure could easily open up the angle and reduce the pressure required to initiate reflux.

These findings were similar to Marchand who, in an animal model, determined that by either accentuating or decreasing the angle one could increase or decrease the pressure required to induce reflux [21]. Removal of the left hemi-diaphragm alone accentuated the angle and required a significantly higher pressure to induce reflux, whereas fundic resection flattened the angle and markedly decreased the pressure requirement. Removal of both diaphragms also resulted in very low native pressure, suggesting that the hiatal canal also plays a significant role in barrier function.

When studied during endoscopy, the valve can be graded according to Hill from grade I–IV [22]. With progressive effacement or shortening of valve length, there is a correlative loss of the valve function which corresponds to increasing Hill grade. This has been shown to be more predictive of the severity of GERD than LES pressure, likely because the Hill grading system reflects the sum total of the four components rather simply measuring LES pressure.

A recent European study [23] looked at the functional anatomy of the flap valve with 3D MRI reconstructions and concurrent high resolution manometry (HRM).

They imaged patients in a fasted state and after a large test meal and found that patients with reflux disease were more likely to have a wider esophagogastric insertion angle with altered gastric morphology. Their EGJ also opens wider and allows for larger volume reflux than in healthy controls. This confirms prior observations and reiterates the complex anatomic geometry that goes into the reflux barrier and that needs to be addressed during any surgical procedure to achieve success.

Crural Diaphragm

Another important component of the reflux barrier is the diaphragm and hiatal canal it creates as the esophagus passes from the low pressure thoracic cavity to the higher pressure abdominal cavity. The exact contribution of the diaphragm on the reflux barrier has been difficult to determine because of its juxtaposition with the LES. Conceptually, the relationship between the crural pillars and the esophagus was likened to the anal sphincter where the rectum passes through sling of the puborectalis muscle [24]. This crural sling around the esophagus is best appreciated when viewed from the abdomen looking up toward the esophageal hiatus and laterally as the esophagus passes through the sling. Removal of the diaphragm, as mentioned above, or its resection entirely, reduces the pressure required to induce reflux considerably [21, 25].

Additional evidence for the role of the diaphragm in barrier function comes from studies of rats and opossums, where the diaphragm and GEJ are spatially separated by a long intra-abdominal esophagus. These animals therefore have two distinct high pressure zones. The first corresponds to the LES and the second is a respiratory-dependent crural component that has comparable pressures [26]. Although this is a distinctively different anatomy than ours, these findings underline a significant crural component to the reflux barrier.

Different modalities have been used to measure the crural component on the LES in humans. Measurement of electrical activity of the crura in healthy controls has shown a linear increase of both electrical activity of the crura and concomitant LES pressures [27]. When HRM is used in patients with documented GERD, they are found to have a significantly greater crural-diaphragmatic (CD) separation compared to patients with functional heartburn or healthy controls [28]. They also have less inspiratory augmentation of their GEJ pressures, again underlying the importance of an intact LES/CD unit in the prevention of reflux.

Phrenoesophageal Ligament

The phrenoesophageal ligament is a suspensory ligament that allows for adequate mobility of the GE junction while retaining its overall relationship to the crural diaphragm, and by doing so, ensures the correct function of the LES/CD unit in preventing reflux. It is the membranous extension of the transversalis fascia and consists of two leaflets, a thicker upper leaflet, and a thinner lower leaflet. Its thickness ranges from 0.8 to 2.3 mm and it can be easily identified as a thickened glistening circular plate that can be freely dissected off the lower surface of the hiatus [29]. The upper leaflet travels up obliquely and inserts into the esophageal wall above the esophageal hiatus. It can penetrate the esophagus and has been found to communicate with the intermuscular septum and the submucosa of the esophagus [30]. The lower leaflet is thought to pass downwards and insert 1–2 cm above the esophageal-gastric angle. As the leaflets degenerate over time, the elastic, collagen, and smooth muscle fibers of the ligament are increasingly replaced with adipose tissue. This progressive change can, in part, explain the rise in incidence of hiatal hernias with increasing age.

The Reflux Barrier in Disease

The fundamental abnormality in the development of GERD is loss of an effective barrier combined with the composition of refluxed gastric contents. The loss of an effective barrier usually occurs over a period of many years. During this time, the normal sphincter undergoes significant changes that lead to worsening reflux and further degradation of the sphincter. This cycle begins with repeated gastric distension causing effacement of the sphincter and LES incompetence, thereby exposing the distal esophagus to chronic reflux [31] and erosion. Over time, this results in progressive scarring, weakening, and shortening of the LES [32]. These factors, together with increasing aerophagia as well as compensatory eating to decrease GERD symptoms, further promote the vicious cycle (Fig. 1.5).

Theoretically, this cycle results in a spectrum of GERD which can range from non-erosive, to mild, moderate, and severe erosive reflux disease, Barrett's dysplasia, and esophageal adenocarcinoma (Fig. 1.6). This evolution is paralleled by progressive barrier dysfunction. Fifty-six percent of non-erosive reflux disease patients (NERD) and 60 % of mild erosive reflux disease (ERD) patients have mechanically defective sphincters, as defined by hypotensive sphincters less than 6 mmHg, shortened LES <1 cm, and shortened intra-abdominal length <2 cm, in comparison to 80 and 77.3 % of patients with severe ERD and Barrett's esophagus [33].

Another mechanism that is associated with gastric distension and reflux are the concepts of LES shortening and transient LES relaxation. Initially, TLESRs were thought to be the reason for reflux occurring. However, TLESRs occur with the same frequency in patients with GERD and healthy controls, though they seem to be more often associated with acid reflux in the diseased population [34]. It's becoming clearer that this complete relaxation of the LES that is not associated with swallowing is normal and occurs as a venting mechanism after gastric distension. More recent data [31] demonstrate that with increasing gastric distension, there is shortening of the LES and with it a subsequent drop in pressure—the transient LES relaxation. This, in part, is thought to be a vasovagal-mediated response to stretch

Fig. 1.5 Cycle of GERD

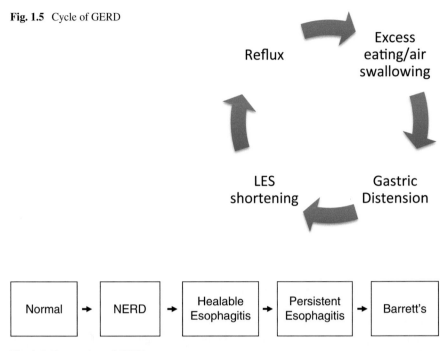

Fig. 1.6 Progression of GERD

receptors in the fundus that lead to relaxation of the LES. Although its contribution toward the pathogenesis of GERD is still under investigation, theoretically, these are the earliest changes leading to deterioration of the reflux barrier that gives way to GERD.

Although GERD's etiology is multi-factorial, obesity is a key component that leads to degradation of the barrier and progressive reflux [35, 36]. The prevalence of GERD is increased for obese patients with a BMI >30 and has been found to be as high as 39 % in a large VA study [36]. This incidence even increases up to 61 % in patients with a BMI >35 [37]. The effects of obesity on the reflux barrier are manifold with morbidly obese patients being twice as likely to have structurally defective LESs than normal controls [35]. A high waist to hip ratio >0.9 was independently associated with long segment BE in White men [38] and central obesity more than doubles the risk for developing BE [39]. Obese patients are also more prone to developing hiatal hernias [40], which in return predisposes them to developing more severe forms of GERD [41, 42].

In terms of the composition of refluxed gastric contents, the concept of a proximal acid pocket has regained popularity. The concept had been originally described over a century ago [43, 44], with the identification of a 2 cm acidic coat that surrounded the proximal gastric contents. This was explained in part by failure of the fundus to mix the chyme due to its decreased peristalsis and reservoir function. Recent studies have identified a region of high acidity at the gastroesophageal junction (GEJ), especially after meals [45]. This appears counterintuitive since food and drink dilute the gastric acid and increase the intra-gastric pH. Some authors have begun to differentiate between trans-sphincteric and intra-spincteric reflux, reasoning that intra-sphincteric reflux may be a more significant culprit in the development of metaplasia and dysplasia. Furthermore, evidence exists that metaplasia and the subsequent dysplasia of the GEJ begins distally and progresses proximally as the LES continues to degrade and efface [46]. It is known that obesity and increased abdominal pressure contribute towards intra-sphincteric reflux [47] and that this effect is even more pronounced in patients with hiatal hernias [48].

Hiatal hernias have been shown to have multiple effects on the reflux barrier that contribute towards GERD and its progression. Although common in the general population, they are frequent in patients with documented GERD and reach rates of 50–94 % [49]. Hiatal hernias lower the LES pressure by separating the intrinsic LES component from the extrinsic crural component and patients with hiatal hernias have shorter LESs in comparison to normal controls [49]. When direct intra-operative measurements of the diaphragmatic hiatus are performed and the hiatal surface area (HSA) is calculated, an inverse correlation between HSA and decreased LES pressures is found. Furthermore, HSA correlates with a significant increase in supine reflux events and overall total reflux events are bordering on significance [50]. Hiatal hernias also lead to decreased esophageal acid clearance, especially in the prone position, and are associated with worsening esophagitis and with a proportional increase in TLESR frequency [51]. Hiatal hernia size is found to be an independent risk factor, along with length of Barrett's disease and severity of reflux, for esophageal adenocarcinoma [42].

Reconstruction of the Reflux Barrier

Reconstruction of a defective reflux barrier is, generally, accomplished through an established anti-reflux operation, which includes a fundoplication. Reconstruction is divided into two steps—crural reconstruction and fundoplication. Initially, crural repair was undertaken to address reduction of the hiatal hernia if present and prevent re-herniation of the repair. Current understanding of reconstructing the reflux barrier suggests that the crural repair plays a greater role in the barrier function than previously understood. In one study, the diaphragm was calculated to be the main determinant of EGJ pressure, whereas the LES was negligible to the overall pressure [52]. Another more specific study quantified intraoperatively the separate contributions of crural closure and fundoplication towards LES pressure and length during Nissen fundoplication. In this study crural closure equally added to LES length and contributed significantly to LES pressure [53]. Furthermore, excessive crural closure also contributes significantly towards persistent dysphagia after fundoplication [54].

Comparatively, fundoplication was only thought to increase LES pressure [55] and restore overall LES length [56]. We now know that fundoplication acts to decrease or impede LES shortening [57] and thus the frequencies of TLESRs. This is accomplished through increasing gastric distension in the wrap, which transmits pressure to the native LES through the fundoplication, thereby preventing it from effacing and thus shortening. In part, this is likely the reason for the more common side effects after fundoplication such as bloating and flatulence.

Lastly, surgical dissection destroys the often faulty suspensory phrenoesophageal ligament, typically without any significant afterthought or effort at reconstructing it. In most antireflux repairs, its destruction is seen as being a necessary step but it's unclear how necessary it really is. Its preservation and potential incorporation in future repairs or treatments may decrease recurrence rates and improve outcomes. For example, newer antireflux options such as magnetic sphincter augmentation, endoscopic fundoplication, and electrical stimulation of the LES all preserve this ligament.

Challenges to Optimal Restoration of the Reflux Barrier

Significant challenges remain for surgeons in reconstructing a functional reflux barrier. It is widely recognized that the long-term effect of fundoplication for a patient with GERD will deteriorate up to 47 % of the time [58]. Although this result is better than optimal medical therapy, this number argues not only for the need for improvement of our surgical therapies and patient selection, but also to better understand this deterioration over time. Failure to break the cycle of large meals and gastric distension may contribute, but there are also structural aspects of the surgical reconstruction that are still in evolution. We have gained insight into improving our repairs from similar deteriorations seen in patients who undergo reconstruction for paraesophageal hernias, where long-term recurrence rates are as high as 57 % [59]. Complete esophageal dissection and adjunct maneuvers such as Collis gastroplasty, intra-abdominal fixation of the GE junction, or crural relaxing incisions have been advocated to decreased recurrence rates and can be employed during fundoplication [60].

When an antireflux repair fails, particularly the Nissen fundoplication, these failures can be categorized into four well-recognized patterns(Fig. 1.7, Table 1.1) [61, 62]. These four patterns are thought to result from failure to address two key forces: axial tension along the esophagus and radial tension on the diaphragmatic hiatus (Fig. 1.8). An additional factor that is not always discussed but merits restatement is repeated gastric distension due to dietary choices and meal sizes. There are virtually no data for fundoplication failure in this area, but experience and extrapolation of data from the bariatric surgeons heightens its importance for future analysis.

Axial tension is thought, at least in part, to be due to esophageal shortening that results from chronic reflux, inflammation, and scarring. The incidence of short esophagus, defined as the inability to restore 2 cm of intra-abdominal esophagus

Fig. 1.7 Types of failure for Nissen fundoplication [63]. With permission: Elsevier, Inc, Southwestern Surgical Congress, et al. Hatch KF, Daily MF, Christensen BJ, Glasgow RE. Failed fundoplications. Am J Surg. 2004;188(6):786–91. Vol 188, Issue 6, 2004, Fig. 1

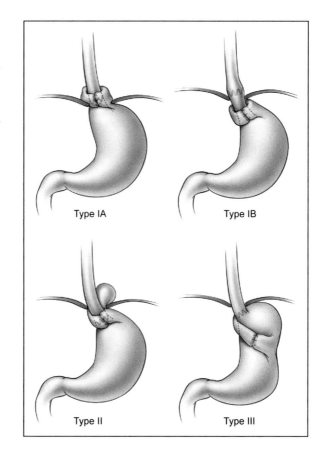

Table 1.1 Patterns of failure (adapted from [61, 62])

Classification	Type I A	Type I B	Type II	Type III
Location of GEJ	Intra-thoracic		Intra-abdominal	
Issue	Migration of wrap	"Slipped" Nissen	Paraesophageal hernia	Wrap around fundus
Wrap	Intact	Disrupted	Intact	Misplaced
Cause	Axial tension	Surgeon experience	Radial tension	Surgeon experience
Frequency (%)	30–80	15–30	16–23	6–10

[63], currently is thought to occur in approximately 10–13 % of patients undergoing laparoscopic antireflux surgery [64, 65]. This may have decreased from the previous pre-PPI—"open surgery" era where short esophagus was encountered frequently and lengthening procedures were more common. Mobilization of the distal esophagus above the inferior pulmonary veins may be necessary to reestablish 2–3 cm of

Fig. 1.8 Different forces
of tension. *Source*: Bradley
DD, Louie BE, Farivar AS,
Wilshire CL, Baik PU, Aye
RW. Assessment and
reduction of diaphragmatic
tension during hiatal hernia
repair. Surg Endosc.
2014;796–804, Fig. 1, page
797, with permission of
Springer Science+Business
Media

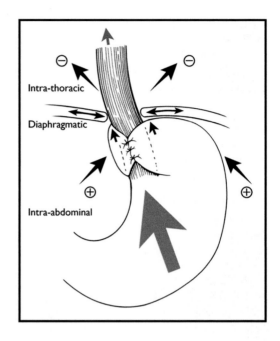

intra-abdominal esophageal length [66]. When an esophageal lengthening procedure is required, there are several options to decreasing axial tension including vagal division [67], Collis gastroplasty [68, 69], or employing a pexy procedure such as the Nissen-Hill hybrid [70], which will be discussed in subsequent chapters.

Other factors potentially contributing to axial tension include the negative pressure of the thorax in conjunction with positive intra-abdominal and intragastric pressure, normal undulation of the GEJ and repetitive contraction of longitudinal esophageal musculature, all combining to place ongoing cephalad stresses on the GEJ and the fundoplication.

Radial tension on the diaphragmatic hiatus until recently has been an under-recognized factor in achieving an optimal repair. Unlike axial tension, which can be approximated by the shortened esophageal length, tension on the hiatus at the time closure has no simple correlate [71]. Assessment has depended on surgeon experience rather than on a quantifiable value. Radial tension may be derived from the shapes or the configurations of the diaphragmatic hiatus—slit, teardrop, "D," and "O". These shapes may also represent a degree of chronicity or progression of the hernia (Fig. 1.9). Few options exist to reduce radial tension, but its recognition may be equally paramount. Both an induced pneumothorax and relaxing incisions appear to change radial tension [71–73]. Whether these maneuvers will reduce recurrence rates remains to be determined.

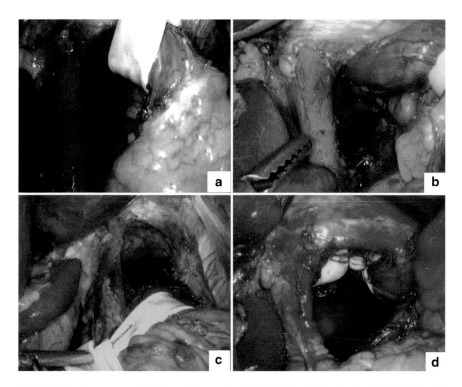

Fig. 1.9 Configurations of the Hiatus. *Source*: Bradley DD, Louie BE, Farivar AS, Wilshire CL, Baik PU, Aye RW. Assessment and reduction of diaphragmatic tension during hiatal hernia repair. Surg Endosc. 2014;796–804, Fig. 3, page 798, with permission of Springer Science+Business Media

Summary

The reflux barrier requires that all of its components act together to prevent reflux, the development of GERD, its progression to Barrett's, and eventually esophageal adenocarcinoma. The proportional contribution of the components towards a functional reflux barrier varies according to patients' anatomy and will be weighted differently according to surgeon training and beliefs. Nonetheless, they require identification and a clear understanding of function in both health and disease in order to address the specific deficits during antireflux surgery to ensure optimal outcomes and prevent further disease progression. Performing a fundoplication is a technical exercise, but performing the right operation correctly on a given patient requires a thorough understanding of the underlying pathophysiology and the anatomic and physiologic components of the reflux barrier and of a successful repair.

References

1. El-Serag HB, Sweet S, Winchester CC, Dent J. Update on the epidemiology of gastro-oesophageal reflux disease: a systematic review. Gut. 2014;63(6):871–80.
2. Cohen E, Bolus R, Khanna D, Hays RD, Chang L, Melmed GY, et al. GERD symptoms in the general population: prevalence and severity versus care-seeking patients. Dig Dis Sci. 2014;59(10):2488–96.
3. Everhart JE, Ruhl CE. Burden of digestive diseases in the United States part I: overall and upper gastrointestinal diseases. Gastroenterology. 2009;136(2):376–86.
4. American Gastroenterological Association. The burden of gastrointestinal diseases. Bethesda: American Gastroenterological Association; 2001.
5. Jackson C. The diaphragmatic pinchcock in so call "cardiospasm". Laryngoscope. 1922;32:132.
6. Forssell G. Studies of the mechanism of movement of the mucos membrane of the Digestive Tract.pdf. Am J Roentgenol. 1923;10(2):87–104.
7. Payne W, Poulton EP. Experiments on visceral sensation. J Physiol. 1927;63:217.
8. Code CF, Fyke FE, Schlegel JF. The gastroesophageal sphincter in healthy human beings. Gastroenterologia. 1956;86(3):135–50.
9. Vantrappen G, Texter EC, Barborka CJ, Vanden-Broucke J. The closing mechanism at the gastroesophageal junction. Am J Med. 1960;28:564–77.
10. Sinnhuber. Beitraege zur Lehre vom muskulaeren Cardiaverschluss. Ztschr klinMed. 1903;50:102.
11. Liebermann-Meffert D. Surgical anatomy of the esophagogastric junction. Helv Chir Acta. 1981;47(6):667–77.
12. Korn O, Stein HJ, Richter TH, Liebermann-Meffert D. Gastroesophageal sphincter: a model. Dis Esophagus. 1997;10:105–9.
13. Stein HJ, Liebermann-Meffert D, DeMeester TR, Siewert JR. Three-dimensional pressure image and muscular structure of the human lower esophageal sphincter. Surgery. 1995;117(6):692–8.
14. Zaninotto G, DeMeester TR, Schwizer W. The lower esophageal sphincter in health and disease. Am J Surg. 1988;155(1):104–11.
15. DeMeester TR, Wernly JA, Bryant GH, Little AG, Skinner DB. Clinical and in vitro analysis of determinants of gastroesophageal competence. Am J Surg. 1979;137(1):39–46.
16. Bonavina L, Evander A, DeMeester TR, Walther B, Cheng SC, Palazzo L, et al. Length of the distal esophageal sphincter and competency of the cardia. Am J Surg. 1986;151(1):25–34.
17. Braune W. Topographisch-anatomisher Atlas nach Druchschnitten an gefrorenen Cadavern. 1878:113–4 p.
18. Von Gubaroff A. Ueber den Verschluss des menschlichen Magens an der Cardia. Arch.fAnat u Physiol. 1886:395.
19. His W. Studien an gehaerteten Leichen ueber Form und Lagerung des menschlichen Magens. Arch Anat u Physiol. 1903;27:345.
20. Thor KB, Hill LD, Mercer DD, Kozarek RD. Reappraisal of the flap valve mechanism in the gastroesophageal junction. A study of a new valvuloplasty procedure in cadavers. Acta Chir Scand. 1987;153(1):25–8.
21. Marchand P. The gastroesophageal spincter and the mechanism of regurgitation. Br J Surg. 1955;42:504–13.
22. Hill LD, Kozarek RA, Kraemer SJM, Aye RW, Mercer CD, Low DE, et al. The gastroesophageal flap valve: in vitro and in vivo observations. Gastrointest Endosc. 1996;44(5):541–7.
23. Curcic J, Roy S, Schwizer A, Kaufman E, Forras-Kaufman Z, Menne D, et al. Abnormal structure and function of the esophagogastric junction and proximal stomach in gastroesophageal reflux disease. Am J Gastroenterol. 2014;109(5):658–67.
24. Allison PR. Reflux esophagitis, sliding hiatal hernia and the anatomy of repair. Surg Gynecol Obstet. 1951;4(92):419–31.

25. Mittal RK, Sivri B, Schirmer BD, Heine KJ. Effect of crural myotomy on the incidence and mechanism of gastroesophageal reflux in cats. Gastroenterology. 1993;105(3):740–7.
26. Soto C, Qi B, Diez-Pardo JA, Tovar JA. Identification of diaphragmatic crural component of gastroesophageal barrier in the rat. Dig Dis Sci. 1997;42(12):2420–5.
27. Mittal RK, Rochester DF, McCallum RW. Electrical and mechanical activity in the human lower esophageal sphincter during diaphragmatic contraction. J Clin Invest. 1988;81(4):1182–9.
28. Pandolfino JE, Kim H, Ghosh SK, Clarke JO, Zhang Q, Kahrilas PJ. High-resolution manometry of the EGJ: an analysis of crural diaphragm function in GERD. Am J Gastroenterol. 2007;102(5):1056–63.
29. Al-Motabagani MAH. An anatomical study of the phrenoesophageal ligament. J Anat Soc India. 2002;51(1):18–22.
30. Kwok H, Marriz Y, Al-Ali S, Windsor JA. Phrenoesophageal ligament re-visited. Clin Anat. 1999;12(3):164–70.
31. Ayazi S, Tamhankar A, DeMeester SR, Zehetner J, Wu C, Lipham JC, et al. The impact of gastric distension on the lower esophageal sphincter and its exposure to acid gastric juice. Ann Surg. 2010;252(1):57–62.
32. Rieder F, Biancani P, Harnett K, Yerian L, Falk GW. Inflammatory mediators in gastroesophageal reflux disease: impact on esophageal motility, fibrosis, and carcinogenesis. Am J Physiol Gastrointest Liver Physiol. 2010;298(5):G571–81.
33. Lord RVN, Demeester SR, Peters JH, Hagen JA, Elyssnia D, Sheth CT, et al. Hiatal hernia, lower esophageal sphincter incompetence, and effectiveness of Nissen fundoplication in the spectrum of gastroesophageal reflux disease. J Gastrointest Surg. 2009;13(4):602–10.
34. Trudgill NJ, Riley SA. Transient lower esophageal sphincter relaxations are no more frequent in patients with gastroesophageal reflux disease than in asymptomatic volunteers. Am J Gastroenterol. 2001;96(9 Suppl):2569–74.
35. Ayazi S, Hagen JA, Chan LS, DeMeester SR, Lin MW, Ayazi A, et al. Obesity and gastroesophageal reflux: quantifying the association between body mass index, esophageal acid exposure, and lower esophageal sphincter status in a large series of patients with reflux symptoms. J Gastrointest Surg. 2009;13(8):1440–7.
36. El-Serag HB, Graham DY, Satia JA, Rabeneck L. Obesity is an independent risk factor for GERD symptoms and erosive esophagitis. Am J Gastroenterol. 2005;100(6):1243–50.
37. Iovino P, Angrisani L, Galloro G, Consalvo D, Tremolaterra F, Pascariello A, et al. Proximal stomach function in obesity with normal or abnormal oesophageal acid exposure. Neurogastroenterol Motil. 2006;18(6):425–32.
38. Kramer JR, Fischbach LA, Richardson P, Alsarraj A, Fitzgerald S, Shaib Y, et al. Waist-to-hip ratio, but not body mass index, is associated with an increased risk of Barrett's esophagus in white men. Clin Gastroenterol Hepatol. 2013;11(4):373–81.e1.
39. El-Serag HB, Hashmi A, Garcia J, Richardson P, Alsarraj A, Fitzgerald S, et al. Visceral abdominal obesity measured by CT scan is associated with an increased risk of Barrett's oesophagus: a case-control study. Gut. 2014;63(2):220–9.
40. Pandolfino JE, El-Serag HB, Zhang Q, Shah N, Ghosh SK, Kahrilas PJ. Obesity: a challenge to esophagogastric junction integrity. Gastroenterology. 2006;130(3):639–49.
41. Howden CW, Henning JM, Huang B, Lukasik N, Freston JW. Hiatal hernia size is the dominant determinant of esophagitis presence and severity in gastroesophageal reflux disease. Am J Gastroenterol. 2001;96(6):1711–7.
42. Avidan B, Sonnenberg A, Schnell TG, Chejfec G, Metz A, Sontag SJ. Hiatal hernia size, Barrett's length, and severity of acid reflux are all risk factors for esophageal adenocarcinoma. Am J Gastroenterol. 2002;97(8):1930–6.
43. Cannon WB. Boston society of medical sciences. Bost Soc Med Sci. 1898;2(6):59–66.
44. Hertz AF. The sensibility of the alimentary canal in health and disease. Am J Med Sci. 1911:132 3.

45. Clarke AT, Wirz AA, Seenan JP, Manning JJ, Gillen D, McColl KEL. Paradox of gastric car-dia: it becomes more acidic following meals while the rest of stomach becomes less acidic. Gut. 2009;58(7):904–9.
46. Chandrasoma PT, Der R, Ma Y, Dalton P, Taira M. Histology of the gastroesophageal junction: an autopsy study. Am J Surg Pathol. 2000;24(3):402–9.
47. Lee YY, Mccoll KEL. Disruption of the gastroesophageal junction by central obesity and waist belt: role of raised intra-abdominal pressure. Dis Esophagus. 2015;28:318–25.
48. McColl KE, Lee TJ. Pathophysiology of gastroesophageal reflux disease. Thorac Surg Clin. 2005;15(3):323–33.
49. Kahrilas PJ, Lin S, Chen J, Manka M. The effect of hiatus hernia on gastro-oesophageal junc-tion pressure. Gut. 1999;44(4):476–82.
50. Koch OO, Kaindlstorfer A, Antoniou SA, Asche KU, Granderath FA, Pointner R. Influence of the esophageal hiatus size on the lower esophageal sphincter, on reflux activity and on symp-tomatology. Dis Esophagus. 2012;25(3):201–8.
51. Kahrilas PJ, Shi G, Manka M, Joehl RJ. Increased frequency of transient lower esophageal sphincter relaxation induced by gastric distention in reflux patients with hiatal hernia. Gastroenterology. 2000;118(4):688–95.
52. Kahrilas PJ, Lin S, Manka M, Shi G, Joehl RJ. Esophagogastric junction pressure topography after fundoplication. Surgery. 2000;127(2):200–8.
53. Louie BE, Kapur S, Blitz M, Farivar AS, Vallières E, Aye RW. Length and pressure of the reconstructed lower esophageal sphincter is determined by both crural closure and Nissen fundoplication. J Gastrointest Surg. 2013;17(2):236–43.
54. Granderath FA, Schweiger UM, Kamolz T, Pointner R. Dysphagia after laparoscopic antire-flux surgery: a problem of hiatal closure more than a problem of the wrap. Surg Endosc Other Interv Tech. 2005;19(11):1439–46.
55. Farrell TM, Smith CD, Metreveli RE, Richardson WS, Johnson AB, Hunter JG. Fundoplications resist reflux independent of in vivo anatomic relationships. Am J Surg. 1999;177(2):107–10.
56. Pandolfino JE, Curry J, Shi G, Joehl RJ, Brasseur JG, Kahrilas PJ. Restoration of normal dis-tensive characteristics of the esophagogastric junction after fundoplication. Ann Surg. 2005;242(1):43–8.
57. Mason RJ, DeMeester TR, Lund RJ, Peters JH, Crookes P, Ritter M, et al. Nissen fundoplica-tion prevents shortening of the sphincter during gastric distention. Arch Surg. 1997;132(7):719–24. discussion 724–6.
58. Lundell L, Miettinen P, Myrvold HE, Hatlebakk JG, Wallin L, Engström C, et al. Comparison of outcomes twelve years after antireflux surgery or omeprazole maintenance therapy for reflux esophagitis. Clin Gastroenterol Hepatol. 2009;7(12):1292–8.
59. Oelschlager BK, Petersen RP, Brunt LM, Soper NJ, Sheppard BC, Mitsumori L, et al. Laparoscopic paraesophageal hernia repair: defining long-term clinical and anatomic out-comes. J Gastrointest Surg. 2012;16(3):453–9.
60. DeMeester SR. Laparoscopic paraesophageal hernia repair: critical steps and adjunct tech-niques to minimize recurrence. Surg Laparosc Endosc Percutan Tech. 2013;23(5):429–35.
61. Richter JE. Gastroesophageal reflux disease treatment: side effects and complications of fun-doplication. Clin Gastroenterol Hepatol. 2013;11(5):465–71.
62. Horgan S, Pohl D, Bogetti D, Eubanks T, Pellegrini CA. Failed antireflux surgery—what have we learned from reoperations. Arch Surg. 2007;134:809–17.
63. Hatch KF, Daily MF, Christensen BJ, Glasgow RE. Failed fundoplications. Am J Surg. 2004;188(6):786–91.
64. Mattioli S, Lugaresi ML, Costantini M, Del Genio A, Di Martino N, Fei L, et al. The short esophagus: intraoperative assessment of esophageal length. J Thorac Cardiovasc Surg. 2008;136(4):834–41.
65. Horvath KD, Swanstrom LL, Jobe BA. The short esophagus: pathophysiology, incidence, pre-sentation, and treatment in the era of laparoscopic antireflux surgery. Ann Surg. 2000;232(5): 630–40.

66. Swanstrom LL, Marcus DR, Galloway GQ. Laparoscopic Collis gastroplasty is the treatment of choice for the shortened esophagus. Am J Surg. 1996;171(5):477–81.
67. Oelschlager BK, Yamamoto K, Woltman T, Pellegrini C. Vagotomy during hiatal hernia repair: a benign esophageal lengthening procedure. J Gastrointest Surg. 2008;12(7):1155–62.
68. Collis JL. An operation for hiatus hernia with short esophagus. Thorax. 1957;12:181–8.
69. Wilson JL, Bradley DD, Louie BE, Aye RW, Vallières E, Farivar AS. Laparoscopy with left chest collis gastroplasty: a simplified technique for shortened esophagus. Ann Thorac Surg. 2014;98(5):1860–2.
70. Qureshi AP, Aye RW, Buduhan G, Knight A, Orlina J, Farivar AS, et al. The laparoscopic Nissen-Hill hybrid: pilot study of a combined antireflux procedure. Surg Endosc. 2013;27(6):1945–52.
71. Bradley DD, Louie BE, Farivar AS, Wilshire CL, Baik PU, Aye RW. Assessment and reduction of diaphragmatic tension during hiatal hernia repair. Surg Endosc. 2015;29(4):796–804.
72. Huntington TR. Laparoscopic mesh repair of the esophageal hiatus. J Am Coll Surg. 1997;184(4):399–400.
73. Greene CL, Demeester SR, Zehetner J, Worrell SG, Oh DS, Hagen JA. Diaphragmatic relaxing incisions during laparoscopic paraesophageal hernia repair. Surg Endosc. 2013;27(12):4532–8.

Chapter 2
Surgical Management of GERD: Recommendations for Patient Selection and Preoperative Work-Up

Sergio A. Toledo-Valdovinos, Kelly R. Haisley, and John G. Hunter

Abbreviations

PPI   Proton pump inhibitors
GERD   Gastroesophageal reflux disease
GI   Gastrointestinal
LES   Lower esophageal sphincter
EGD   Endoscopy or esophagogastroduodenoscopy
BE   Barrett's esophagus
MII   Multichannel intraluminal impedance
CT   Computerized tomography
PUD   Peptic ulcer disease

Introduction

The esophagus plays a vital role in normal digestion, functioning as a conduit for forward passage of foods and liquids to the stomach and gastrointestinal (GI) tract, while simultaneously permitting venting of gaseous contents to facilitate gastric decompression [1]. While there are a multitude of diseases that can affect esophageal function, gastroesophageal reflux disease (GERD) is by far the most common GI tract disorder for which patients seek medical therapy in Western countries [2]. It is estimated that greater than 40 % of the US population experiences occasional GERD symptoms, and as many as 7 % of Americans suffer from daily heartburn [3, 4].

S.A. Toledo-Valdovinos, M.D. • K.R. Haisley, M.D. • J.G. Hunter, M.D. (✉)
Department of Surgery, Oregon Health and Science University,
3181 SW Sam Jackson Park Rd., Mail Code L223A, Portland, OR 97239, USA
e-mail: hunterj@ohsu.edu

© Springer International Publishing Switzerland 2016   19
R.W. Aye, J.G. Hunter (eds.), *Fundoplication Surgery*,
DOI 10.1007/978-3-319-25094-6_2

The result for many is an enormously negative impact on quality of life, creating lifestyle impairments that can be similar in severity to angina or even major depressive illness [3–5]. While GERD is clearly a multifactorial process, the major pathophysiologic cause is a failure of the intrinsic anti-reflux barriers. This can include incompetence of the lower esophageal sphincter (LES), transient sphincter relaxation, insufficient esophageal peristalsis, altered esophageal mucosal resistance, delayed gastric emptying, or altered gastroesophageal anatomy (see Chap. 1). Any one of these conditions, and frequently a combination of several, can incite reflux of gastric contents into the esophagus, leading to bothersome symptoms and potentially long-term complications [2, 6, 7].

While first-line therapy for uncomplicated GERD continues to be medical management with proton pump inhibitors (PPIs), anti-reflux surgery remains an important tool in the stepwise management of the disease, as it addresses the underlying incompetence of the GE junction rather than merely reducing acid production. Although there are multiple potential anti-reflux operations, laparoscopic fundoplication to recreate a competent anti-reflux valve is the mainstay. The goal of this and other anti-reflux procedures is to diminish the volume and/or ameliorate the composition of the refluxate in order to minimize the risks of future complications. Throughout the 1990s, when laparoscopic fundoplication was gaining popularity, there was a sharp rise in the number of anti-reflux procedures performed in the United States, with greater than 30,000 being completed annually [8]. In the years that followed, however, several studies questioned the long-term effectiveness of these operations, citing high rates of resuming medical therapies and poor quality of life outcomes [9]. This, combined with the release of over-the-counter PPIs in the early 2000s, as well as innovations in endoscopic therapies, resulted in a notable decline in the rates of surgical fundoplication, dropping nearly 30 % by 2003 [10]. However, with the improvements in laparoscopic technique and operative experience that have taken place in the last decade, current literature has shown that surgical management is at least equivalent to medications in symptom control and long-term outcomes. Furthermore, in many cases, particularly where medical management has failed, surgical intervention remains the best and most cost-effective option, [11].

Surgical Indications

While the formal indications for anti-reflux procedures have been in flux over the years, surgery is generally justified in patients with GERD symptoms that have been present for an extended period of time (typically greater than 1 year), who have objectively documented reflux (by endoscopy or pH monitoring) and who have failed medical therapy, either through an inability to tolerate medications, or who suffer from persistent symptoms despite adequate medical therapy. This is especially true in cases where the patient's symptoms have a significant impact on quality of life (e.g., spontaneous awakening in the night, interference with physical activity, persistent coughing, or trouble swallowing), or where their reflux is causing health complications, such as aspiration pneumonia, pulmonary fibrosis, asthma, GI bleeding, or esophageal strictures [11, 12]. Such patients stand to benefit significantly from surgical fundoplication and should be evaluated for operative candidacy.

Though medically refractory patients make up the majority of operative candidates, there are additional subsets of patients who may also benefit from surgical therapy. An argument has been made for anti-reflux surgery in patients who have had a good response to medical therapy, but who have severe symptoms when their medications are stopped, indicating that they are likely to require life-long therapy. Studies in these groups have shown a cost benefit to surgical fundoplication over long-term medical therapy [6, 13]. Another unique patient population to consider is those whose refractory symptoms are due to unusual sensitivity of the esophagus, despite a normal amount of acid exposure. This is sometimes called acid hypersensitivity, or functional heartburn. When this condition can be diagnosed (usually using pH and impedance testing to establish a correlation between symptoms and reflux events), it may also predict a successful outcome after anti-reflux surgery [14, 15]. The question of purely elective anti-reflux operations in patients who simply prefer surgery to medications remains somewhat more controversial. It is important to note that despite improving techniques in laparoscopic surgery, there remains a risk for negative impact on quality of life postoperatively. Ultimately, these decisions should be individualized to each patient and provider.

Patient Selection

Given the complexity of GERD, it is paramount that patients who are taken for surgery be carefully screened. As always, proper patient selection is critical to obtaining the best possible surgical outcomes. *While the formal indications for anti-reflux surgery are becoming more concrete, it remains necessary to evaluate each individual patient for their candidacy for surgical intervention.* Unfortunately, neither subjective symptoms nor objective preoperative studies in and of themselves have been shown to predict outcomes following anti-reflux surgery. Rather, overall operative fitness remains the best marker for risk of peri-operative complications. *As would be expected, generally healthy, thin patients with typical symptoms and objectively confirmed reflux have the best surgical outcomes. There are also data to suggest that patients who have been responsive to medical therapy have superior outcomes to those who were only partial responders to medical therapy* [12]. Interestingly, while age does not affect outcomes from surgery [16, 17], there do appear to be differences in results based on gender. Women tend to report worse outcomes compared to men, often describing more symptoms of persistent heartburn and dysphagia, as well as less satisfaction with the overall outcome of surgery. This likely contributes to the higher rate of re-operations seen in the female population [1, 18].

Special consideration must be taken in evaluating patients with GERD and elevated BMIs as obese patients have a higher risk for intra-operative and postoperative complications [11, 19]. Furthermore, in obese patients (BMI >35) with GERD, a traditional anti-reflux procedure may not be sufficient to resolve symptoms. In these cases, bariatric surgery may be a more appropriate option as it can be effective in controlling both obesity and GERD. This comes with the caveat that some bariatric procedures, such as bands or sleeve gastrostomies, can actually provoke or aggravate reflux and should be avoided in overweight patients for whom reflux is already a problem [6, 11, 12].

Psychological disorders and depression may also play a role in the overall success of anti-reflux surgery. As acid secretion and gastric motility can be altered by stress or emotions, psychological disturbances can have a real and measurable impact on acid reflux symptoms for patients both pre- and postoperatively [20]. These patients may have less symptom relief, more postoperative pain, and a lower improvement in quality of life measures after a technically successful anti-reflux surgery, leading to patient dissatisfaction. Whether this is a result of a higher sensitivity of the esophagus (brain–gut axis) or just hypervigilance to symptoms on the part of the patient remains unclear [21, 22].

Ultimately, when any of these risk factors for suboptimal outcomes or lack of response to surgery are identified, a frank discussion about the risks and benefits of proceeding with surgery needs to be held in order to set realistic and achievable expectations for the patient and their outcome postoperatively.

Preoperative Evaluation

Despite its high prevalence, the diagnosis of GERD can present quite a diagnostic challenge due to its often non-specific manifestations and considerable symptom overlap with other conditions such as achalasia, spasm, esophageal cancer, gastritis/PUD, biliary diseases, or even cardiac chest pain [2, 11]. When patients present with a history consistent with typical or uncomplicated GERD, most practitioners are comfortable initiating a trial of antisecretory medications (PPIs or H2 blockers) without the need for a more objective workup of reflux [2, 17]. However, the sensitivity and specificity of making a diagnosis of GERD based solely on clinical presentation is marginal, around 50 % and 70 %, respectively [23]. *Thus, when considering a patient for an anti-reflux operation, symptoms alone are insufficient, and further testing is imperative to definitively confirm the diagnosis of reflux disease prior to proceeding.* This is especially true in patients with atypical symptoms, where a more intense and detailed investigation is needed. Because GERD can affect multiple aspects of esophageal physiology, and surgical approaches vary depending on esophageal function and anatomy, there is no single test that can provide all the essential information. *Thus, a complete, multimodal evaluation is required, which includes a thorough history and physical, upper endoscopy, video esophagram, pH monitoring, and esophageal motility* [4]. *Through the combination of these modalities, and with the adjuvant studies of impedance testing, gastric emptying, and CT when indicated, the preoperative evaluation will document the degree and severity of the reflux, define the esophageal and gastric anatomy, and determine the esophageal function.*

History and Physical

Evaluation of potential surgical candidates starts with a meticulous history and physical examination. In patients with GERD, the history should concentrate on the symptoms of acid reflux and its potential complications. *This should include determining the severity and duration of reflux, coexisting symptoms such as cough, hoarseness, bile regurgitation, nocturnal awakening, and dysphagia, as well as previous or current medications and compliance with and symptom response to those therapies.* While symptoms can sometimes be non-specific, there are often hallmark presentations of the disease. The physical manifestations of GERD can be divided into typical (esophageal) or atypical (extra-esophageal) symptoms. The cardinal typical symptom of GERD is pyrosis (heartburn), a substernal discomfort, or sensation of burning that may radiate upwards towards the neck. Pyrosis is often aggravated by large, fatty meals, though can also be provoked by spicy foods, chocolate, alcohol, or coffee, among other things. Additional typical symptoms of GERD may include regurgitation (the retrograde passage of liquid or food into the mouth or hypopharynx, in the absence of retching or vomiting), dysphagia (subjective difficulty of the passage of food through the esophagus), or non-specific chest pain. The atypical, or extra-esophageal symptoms of GERD, which are more common in the elderly population, include asthma, chronic cough, hoarseness, dental erosions, pharyngitis, sinusitis, idiopathic pulmonary fibrosis, recurrent pneumonia, aspiration, and chronic bronchitis [2, 6, 7, 16, 17]. A less common manifestation of GERD is the phenomenon of "water brash," which is the sensation of salty salivary hypersecretion that is precipitated by the presence of acid in the distal esophagus. Because swallowing of bicarbonate-rich saliva helps to neutralize the acidic pH of the distal esophagus following a reflux event, this mechanism is protective against esophageal damage caused by acid reflux. Patients with impaired salivary function, potentially a result of Sicca syndrome or radiation treatment of head and neck cancers, are missing this important defense mechanism and may be more prone to esophageal complications of reflux disease. *With regard to symptom response to treatment, a very helpful clue suggesting a reflux etiology for both typical and atypical symptoms, a careful history can be clarifying: for example, was the initial response to medical therapy convincing? or if acid suppressants are withheld, e.g., for pH testing, do the symptoms worsen substantially?*

Upper Endoscopy

Upper endoscopy or esophagogastroduodenoscopy (EGD) is the main clinical tool used to evaluate for esophageal complications of GERD, as visualization of the esophageal mucosa allows for a direct assessment of the damage caused by acid reflux [3]. The presence of erosive esophagitis or Barrett's esophagus (BE), both sequelae of acid exposure, is adequate to confirm the formal diagnosis of GERD without further testing, even if pH monitoring has not been completed [4]. In the PPI era, however, altered esophageal mucosa is only present in approximately half of patients with GERD, so a negative study is not sufficient to exclude the diagnosis. It is arguable that while sometimes diagnostic of GERD, the more valuable aspect of EGD is to exclude the presence of an unrecognized esophageal, gastric, or duodenal pathology. This can include BE, which can be present in 10–14 % of GERD patients [23], esophageal strictures, or even underlying dysplasia or cancer. In addition, while the assessment is largely subjective, endoscopy can provide a visual impression of the integrity of the anti-reflux barrier by identifying patulousness of the GE junction, generally associated with a hiatal hernia. Currently, EGD is performed as part of the routine preoperative evaluation in all patients being worked up for an anti-reflux procedure. It is particularly important in individuals with weight loss (usually >5 %), hematemesis, anemia, and/or dysphagia. Endoscopy is also indicated in any patient with risk factors of esophageal cancer or BE, such as family history of BE or esophageal adenocarcinoma, smoking history, obesity, male gender, age >50, white race, or prolonged reflux symptoms [2, 24]. Other indications for preoperative endoscopy include symptoms that are persistent or progressive, despite appropriate medical therapy, evidence of a mass, ulcer, or stricture in other imaging studies, or the need for placement of a wireless pH monitor [24].

Video Esophagram

A video esophagram is a dynamic fluoroscopic evaluation of the esophagus similar to an upper GI study, but with special focus on esophageal anatomy and function. In this study, both video and still images (spots) are obtained which show peristalsis and bolus clearance as well as providing significant anatomical information. This is the best study to determine esophageal length, which can be of great importance in operative planning, as a foreshortened or tortuous esophagus may require an esophageal lengthening procedure or more extensive mediastinal dissection [25]. It is not a reliable study to diagnose gastroesophageal reflux, as esophago-esophageal reflux may be misinterpreted, but it may provide confirmation. Additionally, esophagram is able to show the presence or absence of a hiatal hernia, along with the size and type, which would need to be addressed during an operative repair. Hiatal hernias, particularly those that are large, can be associated with symptom worsening as well as potential complications (e.g., torsion, strangulation, perforation, or massive hemorrhage). When found in conjunction with GERD, hiatal hernias should always be repaired during anti-reflux surgery. However, isolated hiatal hernias can also be an indication for surgery and giant hiatal hernias (type III mixed paraesophageal hernias), whether associated with documented reflux or not, should generally be repaired whenever they are symptomatic (reflux symptoms, post-prandial discomfort, shortness of breath, occult or overt GI bleeding) or when associated with iron deficiency anemia.

Ambulatory pH Monitoring

Currently, ambulatory pH monitoring is considered the gold standard for the diagnosis of GERD. The test is based on objective detection of acid changes in the esophageal lumen and evaluates the number and length of reflux episodes as well as positional components (upright or supine) to generate a composite pH score (the DeMeester score), which is a global measure of the severity of reflux. This can be accomplished by either a trans-nasal catheter left in place for 24 h, or a wireless system (Bravo) that will collect information for 48 h, with the latter being more sensitive to acid exposure by 22 % [3, 4]. Whenever the diagnosis of GERD is in question, such as in cases where patients have normal EGD findings but symptoms consistent with reflux, pH monitoring should be performed during the preoperative work-up. Importantly, the test will be unreliable in a patient who is on PPI therapy, as the acid content of the refluxate will be dramatically reduced by the medical therapy. For this reason, contrary to occasional practice in GI circles, the test should be performed after adequate washout of PPI or antisecretory drugs, which typically requires discontinuation 10 days to 2 weeks before testing [6]. For patients who cannot tolerate discontinuation, impedance pH testing is an alternative (see below).

Esophageal Manometry

Esophageal manometry utilizes intraluminal pressure sensors to garner information on peristaltic coordination, contraction amplitude, and sphincter relaxation of the esophagus. Standard pull-through manometry has recently been replaced by high-resolution esophageal manometry, which utilizes an increased number of pressure probes and integrated impedance testing for data collection. It is faster, easier to perform, and more accurate, capable of providing topographic plotting of esophageal pressure waves and bolus movement [3, 4]. The result is a detailed and accurate assessment of the function of the esophageal body. *While esophageal manometry is not necessary for making the diagnosis of GERD, it is invaluable in its ability to assess esophageal function, which is critical to operative planning (see below).* Manometry data are also important to rule out diseases such as achalasia or scleroderma (which can be easily misdiagnosed for GERD), can demonstrate the presence or absence of hiatal herniation [6], and is important for determination of the optimal placement of the pH probes or impedance catheters [4, 26]. Manometry also provides information on the severity of incompetence of the LES, though ultimately this has little impact in the outcomes of anti-reflux surgery [27].

An understanding of esophageal function by manometry, specifically the peristaltic coordination and strength, is vital to operative planning, as it can greatly impact the type of fundoplication that will be performed. A poor surgical outcome can result when a motility disorder is missed preoperatively, and an aperistaltic esophagus is subjected to a complete fundoplication. This may create a functional obstruction to an esophagus that lacks the coordination or strength to move a bolus past the wrap. The result can be persistent dysphagia, pain, and a potential for re-operation. It has been shown that in comparing patients with normal motility versus those with minor motility disorders, frequently termed "ineffective esophageal motility," dysphagia is no more frequent postoperatively when a total fundoplica-tion is performed compared to a partial wrap [28]. However, when more severe dysmotility is detected preoperatively, a partial wrap is favored over a total fundo-plication with the intent to avoid postoperative dysphagia [4, 6].

Impedance Testing

Multichannel intraluminal impedance (MII) is a technique that provides additional information on the movement of substances through the esophagus. MII functions by detecting changes in resistance to alternating current between two metal elec-trodes placed in the esophagus. As liquid boluses have a very high conductivity, they produce a decrease in the impedance from baseline. Conversely, air, which has a very low conductivity, creates an increase in the impedance from baseline. This way, electrical conductivity differences between the esophageal wall and the esoph-ageal lumen are able to identify the presence of fluid and the air preceding it. By taking different segmental measurements along the course of the esophagus, imped-ance testing can distinguish between antegrade bolus transit (swallow) and retro-grade bolus transit (reflux) [3, 29].

Impedance testing is not used in isolation, but rather in conjunction with pH monitoring, manometry, or both. When used with pH monitoring, as is standard in the Bravo wireless pH detection systems, data obtained from impedance testing offers a supplementary measurement of the severity of reflux that is independent of pH, measuring both acid and non-acid reflux such as bile. When combined with manometry in the current high-resolution manometry devices, it provides valuable information about the effectiveness of liquid transit through the esophagus, which may not have been completely evaluated by pressure measurements alone. Thus, the addition of MII is a useful tool that increases the diagnostic value of both pH testing and esophageal manometry [3, 30], and while it is not routinely necessary, it can be extremely helpful in borderline cases where the results of standard testing are unclear.

Computerized Tomography

Computerized tomography (CT) scans can sometimes be useful in the preoperative evaluation of patents with GERD when concerns for abnormal anatomy exist. Chest and/or abdominal CT may provide valuable information about complex diaphrag-matic hernias or potential masses. Unfortunately, CT is not a good diagnostic test for GERD, due to its static nature, which leads to a low capacity to demonstrate gastric content reflux. Even when gastric reflux is visible on CT, it does not necessarily indicate pathologic or abnormal reflux, and sensitivity and specificity for the diagnosis of GERD are only 40 % and 85 %, respectively [23]. Thus, while CT may be utilized as an adjuvant tool, it is not required for the diagnosis or preoperative evaluation of GERD.

Gastric Emptying Study

While gastric emptying studies are not routinely done as part of the preoperative work-up for anti-reflux surgery, they should be considered in certain patients, namely those with symptoms or risk factors of gastroparesis or gastric dysmotility. More common in diabetic patients, gastroparesis may manifest as persistent abdominal distension, bloating, nausea, or emesis or may be suggested by the presence of retained food in the stomach during EGD despite fasting overnight [4]. It is estimated that up to 20 % of patients with GERD have some degree of gastroparesis, and it is important to recognize that they are at risk of worsening symptoms postoperatively if their gastric dysfunction is not addressed. Physiologically, fundoplication creates a one-way valve at the LES, limiting the natural ability to vent gaseous contents through the esophagus. It is not uncommon for normal patients to experience bloating syndromes following fundoplication due to a failure of proximal decompression, though symptoms are typically mild, as forward motility is preserved. However, when a patient suffers from delayed gastric emptying, the problem of bloating and nausea can be severely compounded.

In mild cases of gastroparesis, fundoplication alone may still be an appropriate surgical option. Postoperative gastric motility studies in patients with known gastric delays have shown that fundoplication alone provides a 38 % improvement in gastric emptying [31]. In more severe cases, pyloroplasty is reasonable to consider, providing an additional benefit by accelerating gastric emptying by up to 70 %, a much greater degree than fundoplication alone [31]. Although there are no specific preoperative gastric emptying cut-off values that necessitate pyloroplasty, the degree of gastric dysfunction in high-risk patients should be formally assessed preoperatively and treatment decisions tailored to the patient's symptoms.

Conclusion

Despite advances in medical therapy, surgical anti-reflux procedures remain a necessary tool in the management of advanced and refractory GERD, with the latest guidelines from the American College of Gastroenterology indicating that, "surgical therapy is as effective as medical therapy for carefully selected patients with chronic GERD when performed by an experienced surgeon (strong recommendation; high level of evidence)" [10]. The comprehensive preoperative evaluation described above helps surgeons to determine which patients are most likely to benefit from surgical intervention and which of the several anti-reflux procedures will suit them best. On completion of preoperative evaluation, the surgeon should be able to discern if the patient's symptoms are compatible with and correlate to the presence of objectively documented pathological reflux (EGD and pH probe) and whether there are any indications of abnormal anatomy or function that would require alterations of surgical approach (UGI and manometry). Armed with this information, patients can be selected and managed appropriately, realistic postoperative expectations can be set, and surgical outcomes can be optimized. An overly strict application of selection criteria will result in disqualification of many patients who may still benefit considerably from fundoplication; on the other hand, bending the rules carries the potential for serious harm to both patient and surgeon and should only be done in the context of a thorough work-up, a holistic assessment of the individual patient, and careful and explicit counseling and informed decision-making regarding risks, realistic objectives, and alternatives.

Disclosure　The authors have nothing to disclose.

References

1. Bredenoord AJ, Smout AJPM. High-resolution manometry. Dig Liver Dis. 2008;40(3): 174–81.
2. Vakil N, Van Zanten SV, Kahrilas P, Dent J, Jones R, Bianchi LK, et al. The Montreal definition and classification of gastroesophageal reflux disease: a global evidence-based consensus. Am J Gastroenterol. 2006;101(8):1900, 1920; quiz 1943.
3. Tutuian R. Update in the diagnosis of gastroesophageal reflux disease. J Gastrointestin Liver Dis. 2006;15(3):243–7.
4. Jobe BA, Richter JE, Hoppo T, Peters JH, Bell R, Dengler WC, et al. Preoperative diagnostic workup before antireflux surgery: an evidence and experience-based consensus of the esophageal diagnostic advisory panel. J Am Coll Surg. 2013;217(4):586–97.
5. Trus TL, Laycock WS, Waring JP, Branum GD, Hunter JG. Improvement in quality of life measures after laparoscopic antireflux surgery. Ann Surg. 1999;229(3):331–6.
6. Fuchs KH, Babic B, Breithaupt W, Dallemagne B, Fingerhut A, Furnee E, et al. EAES recommendations for the management of gastroesophageal reflux disease. Surg Endosc. 2014; 28(6):1753–73.
7. Frazzoni M, Piccoli M, Conigliaro R, Frazzoni L, Melotti G. Laparoscopic fundoplication for gastroesophageal reflux disease. World J Gastroenterol. 2014;20(39):14272–9.
8. Finks JF, Wei Y, Birkmeyer JD. The rise and fall of antireflux surgery in the United States. Surg Endosc. 2006;20(11):1698–701.
9. Spechler SJ, Lee E, Ahnen D, Goyal RK, Hirano I, Ramirez F, et al. Long-term outcome of medical and surgical therapies for gastroesophageal reflux disease: follow-up of a randomized controlled trial. JAMA. 2001;285(18):2331–8.
10. Katz PO, Gerson LB, Vela MF. Guidelines for the diagnosis and management of gastroesophageal reflux disease. Am J Gastroenterol. 2013;108(3):308–28. quiz 329.
11. Eckardt AJ, Pinnow G, Pohl H, Wiedenmann B, Rösch T. Antireflux 'barriers': problems with patient recruitment for a new endoscopic antireflux procedure. Eur J Gastroenterol Hepatol. 2009;21(10):1110–8.

12. Lundell L. Borderline indications and selection of gastroesophageal reflux disease patients: 'is surgery better than medical therapy'? Dig Dis. 2014;32(1–2):152–5.
13. Sarani B, Scanlon J, Jackson P, Evans SRT. Selection criteria among gastroenterologists and surgeons for laparoscopic antireflux surgery. Surg Endosc. 2002;16(1):57–63.
14. Broeders JAJL, Bredenoord AJ, Hazebroek EJ, Broeders IAMJ, Gooszen HG, Smout AJPM. Effects of anti-reflux surgery on weakly acidic reflux and belching. Gut. 2011;60(4):435–41.
15. Jenkinson AD, Kadirkamanathan SS, Scott SM, Yazaki E, Evans DF. Relationship between symptom response and oesophageal acid exposure after medical and surgical treatment for gastro-oesophageal reflux disease. Br J Surg. 2004;91(11):1460–5.
16. Pizza F, Rossetti G, Limongelli P, Del Genio G, Maffettone V, Napolitano V, et al. Influence of age on outcome of total laparoscopic fundoplication for gastroesophageal reflux disease. World J Gastroenterol. 2007;13(5):740–7.
17. Fei L, Rossetti G, Moccia F, Marra T, Guadagno P, Docimo L, et al. Is the advanced age a contraindication to GERD laparoscopic surgery? Results of a long term follow-up. BMC Surg. 2013;13 Suppl 2:S13.
18. Beck PE, Watson DI, Devitt PG, Game PA, Jamieson GG. Impact of gender and age on the long-term outcome of laparoscopic fundoplication. World J Surg. 2009;33(12):2620–6.
19. Hahnloser D, Schumacher M, Cavin R, Cosendey B, Petropoulos P. Risk factors for complications of laparoscopic Nissen fundoplication. Surg Endosc. 2002;16(1):43–7.
20. Biertho L, Sanjeev D, Sebajang H, Antony M, Anvari M. The influence of psychological factors on the outcomes of laparoscopic Nissen fundoplication. Ann Surg Innov Res. 2007;1:2.
21. Kamolz T, Granderath FA, Pointner R. Does major depression in patients with gastroesophageal reflux disease affect the outcome of laparoscopic antireflux surgery? Surg Endosc. 2003;17(1):55–60.
22. Lee SP, Lee KN, Lee OY, Lee HL, Choi HS, Yoon BC, et al. The relationship between existence of typical symptoms and psychological factors in patients with erosive esophagitis. J Neurogastroenterol Motil. 2012;18(3):284–90.
23. Bello B, Zoccali M, Gullo R, Allaix ME, Herbella FA, Gasparaitis A, et al. Gastroesophageal reflux disease and antireflux surgery-what is the proper preoperative work-up? J Gastrointest Surg. 2013;17(1):14–20.
24. ASGE Standards of Practice Committee, Muthusamy VR, Lightdale JR, Acosta RD, Chandrasekhara V, Chathadi KV, et al. The role of endoscopy in the management of GERD. Gastrointest Endosc. 2015;81(6):1305–10.
25. Durand L, De Antón R, Caracoche M, Covián E, Gimenez M, Ferraina P, et al. Short esophagus: selection of patients for surgery and long-term results. Surg Endosc. 2012;26(3):704–13.
26. Katz PO, Menin RA, Gideon RM. Utility and standards in esophageal manometry. J Clin Gastroenterol. 2008;42(5):620–6.
27. Riedl O, Gadenstätter M, Lechner W, Schwab G, Marker M, Ciovica R. Preoperative lower esophageal sphincter manometry data neither impact manifestations of GERD nor outcome after laparoscopic Nissen fundoplication. J Gastrointest Surg. 2009;13(7):1189–97.
28. Strate U, Emmermann A, Fibbe C, Layer P, Zoring C. Laparoscopic fundoplication: Nissen versus Toupet two-year outcome of a prospective randomized study of 200 patients regarding preoperative esophageal motility. Surg Endosc. 2008;22(1):21–30. Epub 2007 Nov 20.
29. Ummarino D, Salvatore S, Hauser B, Staiano A, Vandenplas Y. Esophageal impedance baseline according to different time intervals. Eur J Med Res. 2012;17:1.
30. Del Genio G, Tolone S, Del Genio F, Aggarwal R, D'Alessandro A, Allaria A, et al. Prospective assessment of patient selection for antireflux surgery by combined multichannel intraluminal impedance pH monitoring. J Gastrointest Surg. 2008;12(9):1491–6.
31. Farrell TM, Richardson WS, Halkar R, Lyon CP, Galloway KD, Waring JP, Smith CD, Hunter JG. Nissen fundoplication improves gastric motility in patients with delayed gastric emptying. Surg Endosc. 2001;15(3):271–4.

Chapter 3
Identification and Management of a "Short Esophagus" and a Complex Hiatus

Stephanie G. Worrell, Joshua A. Boys, and Steven R. DeMeester

Introduction

Normally, several centimeters of the distal esophagus and the gastroesophageal junction (GEJ) lie below the hiatus within the abdomen. When the GEJ, the fundus of the stomach, or both migrate into the chest above the hiatus, a hiatal hernia is present. Intrinsic to the repair of a hiatal hernia is the need to bring the GEJ, stomach, and distal esophagus back into the abdomen. However, since 1950, it has been known that in some patients this can be challenging, particularly those with severe gastroesophageal reflux disease (GERD) or a large hiatal hernia. In these patients esophageal shortening can lead to loss of intra-abdominal esophageal length and put tension on the repair of a hiatal hernia. Dr. J. Leigh Collis described a technique in 1957 to address acquired esophageal shortening [1]. His technique, now referred to as a Collis gastroplasty, creates an extension to the esophagus from the high lesser curvature of the stomach. His gastroplasty was done as a transthoracic procedure. Subsequently, several techniques have been described to create a similar gastroplasty using a laparoscopic approach. The laparoscopic management of a short esophagus is challenging, and as a result, there is a tendency by many surgeons to ignore esophageal length and proceed with a standard repair. However, tension is the enemy of any hernia repair, and long-term successful outcomes with hiatal hernia repairs, as for all other abdominal hernias, require addressing tension when encountered.

S.G. Worrell, M.D.
Division of Thoracic Surgery, Department of Surgery, Keck School
of Medicine of the University of Southern California, 1510 San Pablo St Suite 514,
Los Angeles, CA 90033, USA

J.A. Boys, M.D. • S.R. DeMeester, M.D. (✉)
Department of Surgery, University of Southern California,
1510 San Pablo St Suite 514, Los Angeles, CA 90033, USA
e-mail: sdemeester@surgery.usc.edu

© Springer International Publishing Switzerland 2016   31
R.W. Aye, J.G. Hunter (eds.), *Fundoplication Surgery*,
DOI 10.1007/978-3-319-25094-6_3

Identifying the Short Esophagus

Patients at risk for acquired esophageal shortening include those with advanced GERD with esophagitis, stricture, long-segment Barrett's esophagus, a history of sarcoidosis, caustic ingestion, or scleroderma and those with a large sliding or paraesophageal hernia (PEH) [2, 3]. In some reports, patients with a PEH have the highest frequency of a short esophagus [4]. The presence of a foreshortened esophagus in patients with severe GERD is understandable since exposure to refluxed gastric juice causes mucosal injury and can lead to transmural inflammation, fibrosis, and collagen contraction. An esophageal stricture is strongly associated with a shortened esophagus and the need for a gastroplasty. The presence of both a large hiatal hernia (>5 cm) and an esophageal stricture further increases the risk of a shortened esophagus [2]. In addition, a history of a previous failed antireflux procedure with recurrent hiatal hernia should raise suspicion that the length of the esophagus is short. The etiology of esophageal shortening in patients with a PEH is unclear, but may be related to loss of elasticity in the longitudinal esophageal muscle related to chronic loss of intra-abdominal fixation of the GEJ. While any of these histories should increase the suspicion that a patient may have a short esophagus, none are definitive.

The preoperative work-up for any patient presenting with a hiatal hernia or GERD symptoms should include a thorough history and objective studies to understand the relevant pathophysiology. Potentially important objective studies include upper endoscopy, esophageal manometry, 24 or 48-h pH monitoring, and a videoesophagram. The indication for repair of a sliding hiatal hernia is the presence of documented GERD, while for a PEH it is the presence of symptoms. Symptoms in patients with a PEH may be GERD-related, but often consist of shortness of breath or chest discomfort after meals, dysphagia, or the presence of anemia. The objective studies will define the size, type, and reducibility of any hiatal hernia, presence of a stricture or erosive esophagitis, esophageal function, and the presence and severity of increased esophageal exposure to refluxed gastric juice. A foreshortened esophagus can effectively be ruled out when a hiatal hernia fully reduces in barium esophagram, but in any non-reducing hiatal hernia a short esophagus may be present. *Therefore, while objective studies can rule out a short esophagus, none can accurately identify its presence. Instead, a foreshortened esophagus can only be confirmed by the intraoperative inability to reduce the GEJ below the hiatus by 2–3 cm after mediastinal esophageal mobilization and posterior crural closure.*

Management of the Short Esophagus

Although the existence and frequency of a foreshortened esophagus remains debated, failure to obtain an adequate length of intra-abdominal esophagus during hiatal hernia repair has been proposed as a leading cause for reherniation, slippage, or breakdown of the repair [5]. It has been reported that 20–33 % of patients with an inadequate intra-abdominal length will fail after a fundoplication [3]. *The primary method of esophageal lengthening during repair of a hiatal hernia is mediastinal esophageal mobilization.* This mobilization should be taken to the level of the inferior pulmonary veins in most patients. However, if the view is compromised or scarring in the mediastinum from years of severe reflux complicates the dissection, then avoiding injury to a mediasintal structure takes priority over an extra couple of centimeters of esophageal mobilization. Patients with a large hiatal hernia, particularly a PEH, are often kyphotic, and closing the hiatus posteriorly brings the esophagus anterior and adds intra-abdominal length. In order to accomplish a fundoplication without tension, there should be 2–3 cm of intra-abdominal esophagus below the hiatal closure.

The amount of intra-abdominal esophagus during laparoscopic surgery is deceptive since the pneumoperitoneum artificially elevates the diaphragm and gives the appearance of more esophageal length than what is actually present. With deflation of the pneumoperitoneum, the diaphragm descends and some of the apparent esophageal length is lost. Thus, if posterior crural closure and mediastinal esophageal mobilization are insufficient to provide 2–3 cm of abdominal esophagus, esophageal lengthening is recommended.

Our preferred approach for a Collis gastroplasty has been previously published and is based on the wedge fundectomy Collis gastroplasty (WFCG) technique described by Terry and colleagues [6, 7]. Briefly, a WFCG was performed when intra-operatively there was less than 3 cm of intra-abdominal esophagus after mediastinal mobilization and partial posterior crural closure. The WFCG was created with a 52 Fr bougie in place using a 45 mm endo GIA blue load stapler. The goal was to excise as small a wedge of fundus as possible. Given the limitations of articulating endoGIA staplers, we found that in order to excise only a small portion of the fundus, it was necessary to create a star-fish shaped piece of the proximal fundus by successively cutting through the inferior staple line with each successive staple load until a mark approximately 3 cm below the angle of His was reached (Fig. 3.1). The staple-line was not reinforced, but was buried by the fundoplication. A partial Toupet or complete Nissen fundoplication was added to the WFCG in all patients. Importantly, the fundoplication was kept as high on the gastroplasty as possible, preferably at the top near the GEJ. *The importance of this is the fact that the gastroplasty is made from stomach, and acid production by the gastroplasty above the fundoplication can lead to erosive esophagitis in some patients, particularly if there are several centimeters of gastroplasty above the fundoplication* [6, 8].

In our center, the type of fundoplication, partial or complete, is based on the patient's preoperative symptoms and objective test results. In elderly patients, or those with dysphagia, poor motility on high-resolution manometry, or impaired bolus clearance on videoesophagram, a partial (Toupet) fundoplication is preferred. Others are given a complete (Nissen) fundoplication. *It is important to recognize that the gastroplasty tube is aperistaltic. Therefore, bolus transport through the gastroplasty relies on the motility of the distal esophagus above the gastroplasty. Consequently, we are more liberal with the use of a partial fundoplication in patients who have a WFCG added for a shortened esophagus.*

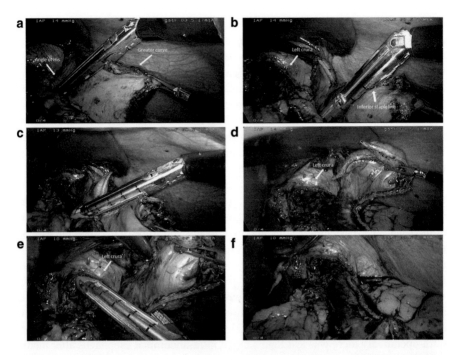

Fig. 3.1 Creation of a wedge-fundectomy Collis gastroplasty with the endo GIA stapler. (**a**) Initial staple line from greater curvature aimed toward the angle of His (**b**) cutting through the inferior staple line gradually working toward mark 3 cm distal to angle of His along lesser curvature (**c**) last staple load is flush against indwelling 52 Fr bougie (**d**) manipulation of the star-fish-shaped piece of the proximal fundus (**e**) stapler now parallel to bougie going up toward angle of His (**f**) final appearance of the Collis staple line with effort made to keep it straight and avoid shark-fin diverticulum at the *top* of staple line

We advocate primary crural closure in all patients given the risk of mesh erosion if the hiatal defect is bridged with synthetic mesh, and hernia recurrence with a biologic or absorbable mesh bridge. *If the crura can't be reapproximated or there is substantial tension on the closure, we use a diaphragm relaxing incision* [9] (see Chap. 4). Typically, we reinforce the primary crural closure with an absorbable (bioabsorbable or biologic) mesh. The use of mesh at the hiatus remains controversial, but in combination with relaxing incisions in the diaphragm and WFCG when indicated, we have had excellent outcomes [10, 11].

Outcome with a Collis Gastroplasty

Before the introduction of laparoscopic surgery, most antireflux procedures were performed in patients with severe GERD, often with impaired esophageal body function. A Collis gastroplasty in these patients frequently led to protracted postoperative dysphagia. In a series reported from our center in 1998, a trans-thoracic Collis gastroplasty in the presence of preoperative dysphagia was significantly associated with a poor postoperative outcome. Many of these patients had strictures and severe reflux disease [12]. The availability of potent acid-suppressing medications has led to a reduction in the acid-related complications of reflux disease including strictures. Furthermore, the number of patients presenting for elective repair of a PEH in the era of laparoscopic surgery is increasing. In these patients, a Collis gastroplasty seems to be better tolerated. In contrast to our earlier series, a recent evaluation of our laparoscopic Collis gastroplasties showed that severe reflux disease was less common. [6] The Collis gastroplasty was done in 72 % of patients either for a PEH or during reoperation for a failed fundoplication. Dysphagia was a common preoperative symptom; however, it resolved in the majority (71 %) postoperatively. Importantly, new-onset dysphagia occurred in only two patients (5.5 %) and resolved after one endoscopic dilatation in both patients. Dysphagia that was present preoperatively and persisted was typically mild and did not significantly impact the patient's diet or lifestyle. The relief of dysphagia in most patients was likely related to repair of the large hiatal hernia and healing of esophagitis. However, we also attributed the low rate of new-onset dysphagia to our "tailored approach" for a fundoplication, using a Toupet rather than a Nissen in patients with manometric evidence of ineffective esophageal motility [6].

A second potential issue with a Collis gastroplasty is acid production by the neoesophagus above the fundoplication. In our recent series, we found that the prevalence of esophagitis after laparoscopic Collis gastroplasty was much lower (11 %) than reported by others. It is not clear why our prevalence was much less than the 36 % rate reported by Jobe et al., but it may in part be related to our efforts to keep the fundoplication as high on the neoesophagus as possible without inducing excessive tension on the repair [13]. It is also possible that the degree of shortening in our patients was less than that in the series by Jobe et al., because in patients with a very short esophagus the Collis gastroplasty can extend above the hiatus. In that circumstance, it is not possible to position the fundoplication at the top of the gastroplasty. Importantly, esophagitis in these patients is often asymptomatic. *Consequently, we recommend that at least one postoperative endoscopy be done after a Collis gastroplasty to evaluate for esophagitis.* If esophagitis is found in the setting of an intact fundoplication, treatment with a proton pump inhibitor is recommended to prevent stricture formation or other complications related to ongoing mucosal injury.

A trans-thoracic Collis gastroplasty has been associated with complications not typically seen with standard antireflux surgery, including staple line leaks, abscesses, and fistulas [14]. *We are always careful to ensure adequate perfusion of the Collis segment and would avoid a Collis gastroplasty if there was any compromise of the lesser curve blood supply due to interruption of the left gastric artery.* In our series of laparoscopic wedge fundectomy Collis gastroplasties, we did not have any of these complications. We routinely cover the Collis staple line with the fundoplication to minimize the risk of a leak or fistula. Further, the wedge fundectomy technique may lead to a wider and more robust portion of fundus that lessens the tension that was sometimes present with a fundoplication after a traditional transthoracic Collis gastroplasty.

The key issue of course with a Collis gastroplasty is whether it reduces hernia recurrence rates. We recently reviewed our experience in 83 patients who had primary laparoscopic PEH repair (manuscript submitted for publication). In 46 patients (55 %), we identified a short esophagus and these patients were given a WFCG. The remainder had a fundoplication alone. At a median follow-up of 9 months, there was objective evidence of a ≥2 cm recurrent hernia in 2 (5.4 %) of the fundoplication alone group compared to 1 (2.2 %) in the WFCG group ($p=0.583$). Two of the three recurrent hernias were small (2–3 cm). The single large recurrent hernia developed in a patient who had a fundoplication alone and required reoperation for recurrent symptoms. Based on this data, one could conclude that a Collis gastroplasty does not alter the frequency of hernia recurrence. However, an alternative conclusion is that without a Collis gastroplasty patients with a short esophagus would have had a higher recurrence rate. If true, then the finding of a similar recurrent hernia rate in patients deemed to have a short esophagus that had a WFCG as we found in those with no esophageal shortening would suggest that addressing a short esophagus is warranted and improves outcomes.

The expected objective hernia recurrence rate after laparoscopic PEH repair is known. The randomized trial by Oelschlager and colleagues reported over 50 % hernia recurrence rate, and the use of biologic mesh did not reduce the rate at 5 years follow-up [15]. Recognizing this high failure rate, which we also reported in 2000, we have modified our approach [16]. It is likely that the high recurrence rate is related to the inherent weakness of the crural tissue and to unaddressed tension on the repair. Tension on the repair of any hernia is a harbinger for failure. *Consequently, we now address lateral tension on the crural closure with a diaphragm relaxing incision and axial tension from a short esophagus with WFCG.* Further, we routinely reinforce the primary crural closure with biologic or absorbable mesh. Using this approach, we have excellent short-term outcomes with a very low objective hernia recurrence rate [10, 11].

Conclusion

Patients found to have a short esophagus during laparoscopic hiatal hernia repair are likely at increased risk for breakdown of the repair and a recurrent hiatal hernia. The first steps to gain esophageal length are mediastinal esophageal mobilization and posterior crural closure. If these steps are inadequate, a Collis gastroplasty should be added. The wedge fundectomy technique allows esophageal lengthening laparoscopically and is associated with a low rate of complications. Clear cut evidence that a laparoscopic Collis gastroplasty reduces hernia recurrence rates is lacking; however, tension on the repair of any hernia is associated with an increased failure rate. Consequently, a Collis gastroplasty in the setting of a foreshortened esophagus is likely to prove beneficial in the long term and should be part of the armamentarium of modern laparoscopic esophageal surgeons.

References

1. Collis JL. An operation for hiatus hernia with short oesophagus. Thorax. 1957;12(3):181–8.
2. Gastal OL, Hagen JA, Peters JH, et al. Short esophagus. Arch Surg. 1999;134:633–8.
3. Horvath KD, Swanstrom LL, Jobe BA. The short esophagus: pathophysiology, incidence, presentation, and treatment in the era of laparoscopic antireflux surgery. Ann Surg. 2000;232(5): 630–40.
4. Herbella FAM, Del Grande JC, Colleoni R. Short esophagus: literature incidence. Dis Esophagus. 2002;15(2):125–31.
5. Hashemi M, Peters JH, DeMeester TR, et al. Laparoscopic repair of large type III hiatal hernia: objective followup reveals high recurrence rate. J Am Coll Surg. 2000;190(5):553–61.
6. Zehetner J, Demeester SR, Ayazi S, et al. Laparoscopic wedge fundectomy for collis gastroplasty creation in patients with a foreshortened esophagus. Ann Surg. 2014;260(6):1030–3.
7. Terry ML, Vernon A, Hunter JG. Stapled-wedge Collis gastroplasty for the shortened esophagus. Am J Surg. 2004;188(2):195–9.
8. Swanstrom LL, Marcus DR, Galloway GQ. Laparoscopic Collis gastroplasty is the treatment of choice for the shortened esophagus. Am J Surg. 1996;171(5):477–81.
9. Greene CL, DeMeester SR, Zehetner J, et al. Diaphragmatic relaxing incisions during laparoscopic paraesophageal hernia repair. Surg Endosc. 2013;27(12):4532–8.
10. Alicuben ET, Worrell SG, DeMeester SR. Impact of crural relaxing incisions, collis gastroplasty, and non-cross-linked human dermal mesh crural reinforcement on early hiatal hernia recurrence rates. J Am Coll Surg. 2014;219(5):988–92.
11. Alicuben ET, Worrell SG, DeMeester SR. Resorbable biosynthetic mesh for crural reinforcement during hiatal hernia repair. Am Surg. 2014;80(10):1030–3.
12. Ritter MP, Peters JH, DeMeester TR, et al. Treatment of advanced gastroesophageal reflux disease with Collis gastroplasty and Belsey partial fundoplication. Arch Surg. 1998;133(5): 523–8; discussion 528–9.
13. Jobe BA, Horvath KD, Swanstrom LL. Postoperative function following laparoscopic Collis gastroplasty for shortened esophagus. Arch Surg. 1998;133(8):867–74.
14. Patel HJ, Tan BB, Yee J, et al. A 25-year experience with open primary transthoracic repair of paraesophageal hiatial hernia. J Thorac Cardiovasc Surg. 2004;127(3):843–9.
15. Oelschlager BK, Petersen RP, Brunt LM, et al. Laparoscopic paraesophageal hernia repair: defining long-term clinical and anatomic outcomes. J Gastrointest Surg. 2012;16(3):453–9.
16. Hashemi M, Peters JH, DeMeester TR, et al. Laparoscopic repair of large type III hiatal hernia: objective follow-up reveals high recurrence rate. J Am Coll Surg. 2000;190(5):553–60.

Chapter 4
Difficult Diaphragmatic Closure

Robert B. Yates, Brant Oelschlager, and Andrew Wright

Introduction

Closure of the esophageal hiatus is a key step in laparoscopic hiatal hernia repair. Approximating the diaphragmatic crura recreates a major component of the antireflux barrier by restoring the normal relationship between the diaphragmatic crura, esophagus, and gastroesophageal junction. Restoring these components of the lower esophageal sphincter contributes to the creation of an antireflux mechanism that prevents gastroesophageal reflux. Additionally, closure of the esophageal hiatus establishes a barrier to prevent a recurrent hiatal hernia (see Chap. 1).

Despite adequate closure of the esophageal hiatus at the time of laparoscopic hiatal hernia repair, recurrent hiatal hernia is common. In one multicenter randomized study, recurrent hernias occurred in >50 % of patients at 5 years following laparoscopic paraesophageal hernia repair [1]. Although the most common symptom associated with a recurrent hiatal hernia is heartburn, fortunately, recurrent hiatal hernias are frequently asymptomatic. While recurrent symptoms of gastroesophageal reflux are frequently manageable with proton pump inhibitor therapy, recurrent hiatal hernias can lead to significant dysphagia or other complications that can require reoperation.

The presence of tension at the esophageal hiatus during hernia repair is thought to be a contributing factor to the development of recurrent hiatal hernia [2]. Consequently, it is important to achieve a tension-free closure of the esophageal hiatus. In the majority of patients, the diaphragmatic crura can be closed

R.B. Yates, M.D. • B. Oelschlager, M.D. • A. Wright, M.D. (✉)
Department of Surgery, University of Washington,
1959 NE Pacific St., 356410, Seattle, WA 98115, USA
e-mail: awright2@uw.edu

© Springer International Publishing Switzerland 2016
R.W. Aye, J.G. Hunter (eds.), *Fundoplication Surgery*,
DOI 10.1007/978-3-319-25094-6_4

primarily under little or no tension (i.e., posterior hiatoplasty). However, when the diaphragmatic crura lack pliability, primary tension-free closure of the hiatus may not be possible. In extreme cases, the crura are so non-compliant that the hiatus cannot be closed.

When faced with a challenging diaphragmatic closure, surgeons have several options: (1) Use mesh or an autologous tissue flap (e.g., falciform ligament or left triangular ligament) to reinforce the hiatal closure under tension or bridge the hiatus if it cannot be closed; (2) Create diaphragmatic (crural) relaxing incisions or an intentional pneumothorax to reduce hiatal tension and facilitate primary closure of the hiatus; or (3) Perform a gastropexy without closure of the hiatus. Importantly, not all these options are created equal. In this chapter, we will elaborate on these techniques and provide a review of the current evidence for their use.

Various types of mesh have been used to reinforce primary hiatal closure [3–5]. *The placement of permanent synthetic mesh at the esophageal hiatus is associated with significant complications, including esophageal stenosis and erosion, and therefore its use in this capacity cannot be recommended* [6–8]. Compared to permanent synthetic mesh, biologic mesh is considered to have a better safety profile at the esophageal hiatus [9]; however, complications have also been reported with biologic mesh reinforcement of crural closure [10]. The evidence that biologic mesh reduces the incidence of recurrent hiatal hernia is mixed: At short-term follow-up (6 months postoperatively), two randomized studies evaluated three different types of biologic mesh reinforcement of posterior hiatoplasty and demonstrated reduced rates of recurrent hiatal hernia compared to primary closure of the esophageal hiatus [11, 12]. At 5-year follow-up, however, biologic mesh did not reduce the rate of recurrent hiatal hernia compared to primary hiatal closure [1].

Autologous tissues are an alternative to synthetic and biologic mesh to buttress primary crural closure or bridge the hiatus if it cannot be closed. Van Helsdingen [13] was the first to report the use of the falciform ligament to reduce the risk of recurrent hiatal hernia. Since then, several studies have investigated the application of autologous tissues to reinforce the hiatal closure or bridge the hiatus. Despite no long-term clinical outcomes studies to evaluate these techniques, autologous tissue repairs are appealing, because they use the patient's own tissues, require minimal additional time to perform, and do not increase the cost of laparoscopic hiatal hernia repair.

The major drawback of any reinforcement of the hiatus is that it does not correct the underlying cause of difficult diaphragmatic closure: hiatal tension. To address this issue, several techniques have been developed. Intentional pneumothorax has been shown to reduce tension at the hiatus during repair [14], but this can lead to temporary hemodynamic instability and compromised oxygenation, and the durability of this technique is unknown. In addition, it is a temporary relief of hiatal tension that will be lost when the capnothorax is resolved. Diaphragmatic (crural) relaxing incisions are another technique to reduce hiatal tension. In general, relaxing incisions facilitate the approximation of two pieces of tissue with little or no tension. Historically, this technique has been applied to primary tissue repair of inguinal hernias (e.g., McVay repair); [15] more recently, relaxing incisions are used to achieve primary closure of the linea alba during repair of large ventral hernias [16]. Diaphragmatic relaxing incisions objectively reduce hiatal tension [14] and can facilitate primary closure of the esophageal hiatus. Finally, when the esophageal hiatus is truly un-closable due to extreme size or elevated tension, laparoscopic gastropexy can relieve esophageal and gastric obstructive symptoms and prevent gastric volvulus without the need to primarily close the hiatus.

The goals of this chapter are to describe the contributing factors to difficult diaphragmatic closure with a particular emphasis on radial tension at the esophageal hiatus and to provide surgeons an in-depth critical review of advanced techniques to manage difficult hiatal closure.

Tension at the Esophageal Hiatus

Two Types of Tension: Axial and Radial

Tension at the esophageal hiatus occurs in two major forms. Axial tension is the force directed parallel to the long-axis of the esophagus. This tension develops from adhesions between mediastinal structures (including the pleurae, aorta, and pericardium) and the hiatal hernia sac, stomach, and esophagus. Clinically, this force pulls the gastroesophageal junction cephalad from the abdominal cavity into the posterior mediastinum. At the time of hiatal hernia repair, axial tension is reduced by mobilizing the esophagus in the posterior mediastinum. *Adequate mobilization is achieved when the gastroesophageal junction lies at least 3 cm below the hiatus.* When posterior mediastinal mobilization fails to obtain adequate intra-abdominal esophageal length, esophageal lengthening procedures can be performed, including vagotomy, Collis gastroplasty, and wedge gastroplasty [17–20] (see Chap. 3).

Radial tension at the esophageal hiatus is directed perpendicular to the long-axis of the esophagus, parallel to the diaphragmatic crura and away from the midline. This force must be overcome to close the esophageal hiatus. Hiatal closure is necessary to reestablish the antireflux mechanism of the lower esophageal sphincter and decrease the risk of recurrent hiatal hernia. In the presence of elevated radial tension, primary closure of the esophageal hiatus can be difficult, if not impossible. Although radial tension is the major factor that prevents hiatal closure during laparoscopic hiatal hernia repair, until recently the specific factors that contribute to increased radial tension at the esophageal hiatus were unknown.

Contributing Factors to Radial Tension at the Esophageal Hiatus

In the most comprehensive evaluation of hiatal tension to date, Bradley et al. [14] investigated the anatomic factors that contribute to radial tension at the hiatus. The authors prospectively identified 50 patients undergoing laparoscopic hiatal hernia repair. All patients underwent preoperative esophagram, and the hernia volume was measured. Additionally, the hernia was classified as ellipsoid (i.e., paraesophageal hernia) or cylindrical (i.e., sliding hiatal hernia).

Intraoperatively, the authors classified the shape of the hiatus according to slit, teardrop, "D," or oval. After complete hiatal dissection and mobilization of the esophagus in the posterior mediastinum, a novel calibrated tension gage (BPI Medical, Fife, WA) was used to measure radial tension at the esophageal hiatus. The results of this study showed a positive correlation between radial tension and width of the hiatus ($r^2 = 0.31$), hiatal surface area ($r^2 = 0.37$), ellipsoid-shaped (paraesophageal) hernia ($r^2 = 0.40$), as well as "D"- and teardrop-shaped hiatus ($r^2 = 0.35$ and $r^2 = 0.45$, respectively), but not for oval- ($r^2 = 0.02$) and slit- ($r^2 = 0.00008$) shaped hiatus. Other patient factors failed to show a positive correlation with radial tension, including patient age and BMI, presence of esophagitis, endoscopic hernia size, cylindrical shaped hernia, and volume of a type I (sliding) hiatal hernia. These results corroborate our experience with challenging hiatal closure during laparoscopic hiatal hernia repair. Specifically, hiatal width alone does not predict the force required to close the hiatus: Some very widely spaced crura are easily approximated, while some which are narrower require dramatically greater force—or may be impossible—to close.

All of the patients in aforementioned study underwent repair of first-time hiatal hernias. To date, no study has assessed tension at the hiatus in patients undergoing repair of recurrent hiatal hernia. However, in our experience at the Center for Esophageal and Gastric Surgery at the University of Washington, a high-volume gastroesophageal surgery program, previous operations at the hiatus appear to be associated with increased radial hiatal tension. If this is true, surgeons would be expected to employ operative techniques that reduce hiatal tension more frequently in reoperative patients. Diaphragmatic relaxing incisions objectively reduce radial tension at the esophageal hiatus, and *in our experience, relaxing incisions were performed nearly twice as frequently in patients undergoing recurrent hiatal hernia repair compared to patients undergoing primary paraesophageal hernia repair (15/138 [11 %] vs. 14/230 [6 %])*. This finding provides indirect evidence that radial tension is higher in reoperative hiatal hernia repair compared to first-time hiatal hernia repair and suggests that hiatal scarring is a contributing factor to radial tension at the esophageal hiatus. However, a prospective study is needed to objectively measure intraoperative hiatal tension in this patient population.

Operative Management of Difficult Diaphragmatic Closure

There are four fundamental maneuvers to manage difficult diaphragmatic closure. First, *primary hiatal closure can be reinforced* with synthetic mesh, biologic mesh, or autologous tissue flaps (e.g., falciform ligament and left triangular ligament). Second, when the hiatus cannot be closed, the *unclosed hiatus can be bridged* using these same materials. Third, diaphragmatic relaxing incisions and intentional pneumothorax can be used to *reducehiatal tension* to achieve primary closure. Finally, when the hiatus is very large and completely un-closable, *gastropexywithout hiatal closure* can correct esophageal obstructive symptoms and prevent gastric volvulus. Use of mesh in laparoscopic hiatal hernia repair has been extensively reviewed elsewhere [5, 9, 21, 22]. In this chapter, we will focus on autologous tissue flaps, diaphragmatic relaxing incisions, intentional pneumothorax, and gastropexy as techniques to address difficult diaphragmatic closure.

Autologous Tissue Flaps

Vascularized pedicle flaps can be used to reinforce primary closure of the esophageal hiatus or create a tissue bridge to cover an unclosable hiatus. The two structures that can be used in this capacity are the falciform ligament and left triangular ligament of the liver.

Falciform Ligament

Table 4.1 summarizes the studies that have evaluated the use of the falciform ligament as hiatal reinforcement or hiatal bridging.

Varga et al. [23] described their technique to reinforce primary closure of the hiatus with the falciform ligament during laparoscopic hiatal hernia repair. After primary closure of the diaphragmatic crura, an ultrasonic dissector is used to release

Table 4.1 Studies of autologous tissue reinforcement of hiatus in patients undergoing laparoscopic Hiatal hernia repair

Study	Tissue used	Study design	N	Mean follow-up	Recurrence	Complications
Laird et al. [25]	Falciform	Prospective, non-randomized	34	7.1 months	9 % (barium swallow); 1 reoperation	6 % (2/34)
Park et al. [26]	Falciform	Case series	15	NR	0 %[a]	0 %
Varga et al. [24]	Falciform	Case series	26	35 months	15 % (barium swallow); 1 reoperation	11.5 %
Varga et al. [23]	Falciform	Case series	4	8.25 months [6–11]	0 % (barium swallow)	0 %
Ghanem [27]	Left triangular	Case series	4	1 year	0 %[a]	0 %

NR not reported
[a]No clinical recurrences, but no systematic follow-up performed

the falciform ligament from the parietal peritoneum. Particular care is taken to preserve the blood supply and prevent hematoma formation. After the ligament is mobilized, it is rotated under the left lateral section of the liver and passed posterior to the esophagus to lie across the closed esophageal hiatus. Four permanent sutures secure the falciform to the right and left crura to create a U-shaped reinforcement of the hiatus.

The results of mid-term follow-up included 26 patients underwent falciform ligament reinforcement of the hiatus during laparoscopic repair of primary ($n=20$) and recurrent ($n=6$) hiatal hernia [24]. Conversion to an open operation was required in all six patients with recurrent hiatal hernias. Three (11.5 %) perioperative complications occurred (pneumothorax, superficial wound infection, and subphrenic abscess). Mean length of stay was 7.4 days (range 4–30). Mean clinical and radiographic follow-up was 35 months (range 17–50 months). Two patients (8 %) reported symptoms of recurrent gastroesophageal reflux; however, 24-h pH monitoring and esophagram were normal. Four patients (15 %) were found to have recurrent hiatal hernias on esophagram, and two of these patients were symptomatic. Three recurrences were in patients who originally had hiatal hernia ≥9 cm, and one recurrence was in a patient who originally underwent recurrent hiatal hernia repair. Only one patient required reoperation due to symptoms that were recalcitrant to medical therapy.

Laired et al. [25] completed the most comprehensive study on use of the falciform ligament during hiatal hernia repair. In 34 consecutive patients who underwent hiatal hernia repair, primary closure of the hiatus was achievable in 32 patients, and the falciform ligament was used to reinforce hiatal closure. In two patients, the hiatus was unable to be closed, and the falciform ligament was used as an autologous tissue bridge to cover the unclosed hiatus. All operations were performed laparoscopically. Thirty-three patients (97 %) completed clinical and radiographic follow-up at mean of 7.1 months. Compared to preoperative scores, significant improvement was seen postoperatively in frequency and severity of the overall symptom score, which assessed ten common gastroesophageal symptoms. On barium esophagram, three patients (9 %) were identified to have a recurrent hiatal hernia. One of these patients reported significant epigastric pain and regurgitation, and reoperative hiatal hernia repair was performed.

Park et al. [26] described their application of the falciform ligament as an autologous tissue bridge when the hiatus was unable to be closed due to excessive radial tension. In their study, due to excessive radial tension at the hiatus, no patient underwent complete primary closure of the hiatus. In these patients, the surgeon created a falciform ligament bridge to cover the portion of the hiatus that remained open. In 15 patients who underwent this operation, no patients required postoperative interventions related to the hiatal hernia repair. Two patients who underwent this procedure required laparoscopy for unrelated reasons, and in each case, the falciform ligament repair appeared intact without evidence of recurrent hiatal hernia. The major weaknesses of this study are its small sample size and the lack of routine postoperative imaging to assess for recurrent hiatal hernia.

In summary, use of falciform ligament appears to be a safe technique to reinforce, or bridge, the hiatus. Short-term follow-up appears good; however, without comparison studies with another closure method, it is difficult to determine whether this technique will reduce recurrent hiatal hernia at long-term follow-up.

Left Triangular Ligament

Gahnem et al. [27] reported the only study of hiatal reinforcement with the left triangular ligament. Their technique begins with standard laparoscopic hiatal hernia repair, and in their experience, posterior closure was achievable in all patients. However, following posterior hiatoplasty, some patients demonstrated an anterior hiatal defect. In these patients, a 54-Fr bougie was placed in the esophagus, and if the size of the residual defect was large enough, the left triangular ligament was mobilized and used to patch the anterior hiatal defect.

In this small series, four patients underwent left triangular ligament coverage of an anterior hiatal defect. The average hiatal defect size was 5.5 cm (range 3–8 cm). No perioperative complications occurred. On postoperative day 1, an esophagram was performed, and no evidence of recurrent hiatal was present in these four patients at that time; however, no intermediate or long-term radiographic evaluation was completed. At 1-year clinical follow-up, there was no evidence of recurrent hiatal hernia; however, the authors do not state their assessment criteria.

From this small case series, left triangular ligament patch of the anterior hiatal defect appears safe. However, before this technique is widely adopted, additional studies are needed in which long-term systematic clinical and radiographic follow-up are performed.

Methods to Reduce Hiatal Tension

Primary repair of hernias is frequently accompanied by tension, and tension is associated with poor outcomes during all types of hernia repairs. Tension at the esophageal hiatus can be addressed with two operative techniques: Creation of an intentional pneumothorax and diaphragmatic relaxing incisions. Bradley et al. [14] first described the creation of an intentional left pneumothorax as a relaxing maneuver. This technique was based on the observation that the left crus becomes more compliant after incidental pneumothorax. Indeed, the results of their study demonstrate objective reduction in hiatal tension with the creation of an intentional pneumothorax.

More commonly, relaxing incisions may be used to reduce tension during hernia repair. By creating an incision in healthy tissue away from the edge of the hernia defect, the hernia edges mobilize to achieve a tension-free primary closure of the hernia. For decades, relaxing incisions were used in the repair of inguinal hernias [15, 28], and more recently, they have garnered enthusiasm among surgeons in the management of large ventral hernias [29, 30].

Nearly 20 years ago, Huntington [31] first reported diaphragmatic relaxing incisions as a method to facilitate primary closure of the esophageal hiatus. Huntington's operative technique for relaxing incisions is particularly appealing, because it facilitates closure of large hiatal defects and allows the use of synthetic mesh reinforcement of the hiatus by leaving a cuff of diaphragm between the mesh and the esophagus. Despite these advantages, crural relaxing incisions have only recently garnered enthusiasm among gastroesophageal surgeons. One reason for the delay in adoption of relaxing incisions into clinical practice was the advent of biological mesh. Early experience with biologic mesh suggested improved safety over synthetic mesh [9] and reduced rates of recurrent hiatal hernia compared to primary hiatal closure alone [12]. However, it is now known that biologic mesh does not reduce the long-term risk of recurrent hiatal hernia [1], and surgeons are reevaluating diaphragmatic relaxing incisions as a method to address difficult diaphragmatic closure and reduce the long-term rate of recurrent hiatal hernia.

The purpose of this section is threefold: First, we discuss the important technical aspects of creating crural relaxing incisions. Second, we review the evidence that intentional pleurotomy and crural relaxing incisions reduce tension at the esophageal hiatus. Finally, we present the available literature that assesses the clinical outcomes of relaxing incisions during difficult diaphragmatic closure.

Diaphragmatic Relaxing Incisions: Operative Technique

During laparoscopic repair of complex hiatal hernias, relaxing incisions are created immediately prior to closure of the esophageal hiatus. Currently, there is no commercially available device to objectively measure hiatal tension, nor is the level of tension at which relaxing incisions confer a clinical benefit known. As a result, the decision to create a relaxing incision is based on the surgeon's subjective assessment of radial tension at the hiatus and, ultimately, the inability to primarily close the hiatus without excessive tension. Intraoperatively, excessive tension is identified as tearing, or imminent tearing, of the crural muscle fibers when the hiatus is approximated with interrupted sutures.

Relaxing incisions are created using electrocautery or ultrasonic energy devices. We use electrocautery to open the peritoneum overlying the diaphragmatic muscle. Using blunt dissection, the crural muscle fibers are separated to expose the underlying pleura. *We avoid creating a full-thickness diaphragmatic incision, as we have found that opening the diaphragmatic peritoneum alone sufficiently mobilizes the crus to allow primary closure of the hiatus without tension, and a full-thickness incision confers no additional benefit.* In addition, a full-thickness relaxing incision opens the pleura, and the pneumothorax that develops can cause hemodynamic instability and/or compromised oxygenation and ventilation of the patient.

The relaxing incision should be made long enough to reduce tension at all points along the hiatus. Generally, the length of the incisions should mirror the length of the hiatus in an anterior–posterior dimension. In our experience, however, the posterior aspect of the hiatus can generally accommodate one or two crural sutures to

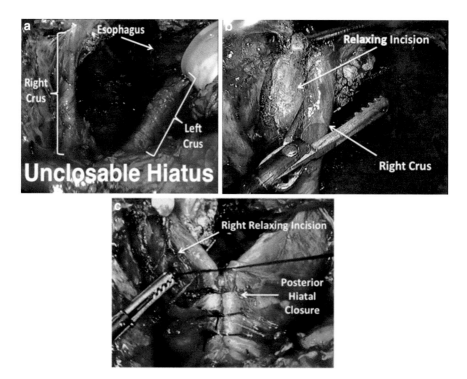

Fig. 4.1 Intraoperative images demonstrating (**a**) an unclosable hiatus; (**b**) the creation of a right crural relaxing incision; and (**c**) the posterior closure of the hiatus after right crural relaxing incision

achieve primary closure of that portion of the hiatus without significant tension (Fig. 4.1). Additionally, the aorta and thoracic duct lie in close proximity to the posterior aspect of the hiatus and are at risk of injury when the incision is extended into this region. Consequently, careful attention should be paid when extending the relaxing incision along this portion of the hiatus.

Laterality of the Relaxing Incision

When a difficult diaphragmatic closure is encountered and a relaxing incision is chosen to facilitate tension-free hiatal closure, one must decide which crus to incise. There is no evidence to suggest the efficacy of a relaxing incision is crus-dependent, and a unilateral incision is sufficient to allow primary tension-free closure of the hiatus in the majority of difficult diaphragmatic closures. The primary factor that determines laterality of the relaxing incision is patient safety.

Complications can occur from the creation of a relaxing incision on either crus: On the left, the phrenic nerve can be transected and result in diaphragmatic paralysis;

on the right, injury to the inferior vena cava can cause devastating hemorrhage. These complications can be avoided by following a few basic principles. *When creating a right-sided incision, adequate distance must exist between the right crural edge and the inferior vena cava. We strive to create the relaxing incision approximately 1–2 cm from the crural edge, as a thinner pillar of crural tissue increases the likelihood of tearing the diaphragm with primary closure. When the right crus is particularly diminutive due to extensive fibrosis or thinned diaphragmatic muscle, or when insufficient distance exists between the crural edge and the inferior vena cava, we place the relaxing incision on the left crus. When creating a left-sided relaxing incision, careful attention must be paid to avoid transecting the phrenic nerve. Two options are available to do this: Either left incision should be created parallel to the seventh rib, as described by Green et al. [32], or medial to the phrenic nerve and close to the hiatus.*

We preferentially create a right-sided relaxing incision to facilitate closure, because it is rare that the right crus will not accommodate a relaxing incision and it is impossible to identify the left phrenic nerve intraoperatively, which increases the risk of inadvertent injury. In addition, by placing the relaxing incision on the right crus, biologic mesh can be used to cover the relaxing incision and reinforce theposterior hiatoplasty (further discussion in next section); when the incision is placed on the left crus, permanent synthetic mesh should be used to patch the incision. If a right-sided incision does not facilitate hiatal closure, we create bilateral relaxing incisions.

Use of Mesh to Reinforcement Diaphragmatic Relaxing Incisions

After a relaxing incision is performed and posterior crural sutures are placed to close the hiatus primarily, the relaxing incision and posterior hiatoplasty should be covered with mesh. When a right-sided incision is created, we use biologic mesh to do this. The mesh is cut into a "C" shape and positioned at the hiatus (Fig. 4.2). Several permanent sutures are placed to attach the mesh to the diaphragm; then the mesh is reflected anteriorly to expose the hiatal closure. With the hiatal closure exposed, fibrin glue is then placed to cover the hiatal closure and the mesh (Figs. 4.2 and 4.3). We have seen no complications with the use of biologic mesh in this capacity.

Early in our experience with crural relaxing incisions, we also used biologic mesh to patch relaxing incisions on the left hemidiaphragm. However, two patients who underwent this procedure developed symptomatic diaphragmatic hernias at the site of the relaxing incision (Fig. 4.4). We did not anticipate this outcome for two reasons: first, we performed left-sided relaxing incisions without breeching the pleura. As a result, the biologic mesh was in direct contact with the fibroadipose tissue of the diaphragm as well as the pleura, and we believed that tissue remodeling would create a barrier to prevent a symptomatic hernia. Second, we created left-sided incisions on the posterior aspect of the left crus, an area that we believed would be protected from herniation of the viscera even if a full-thickness diaphrag-

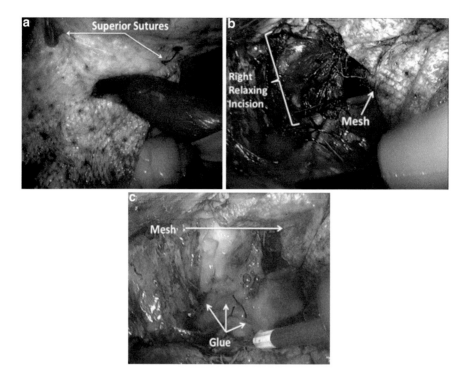

Fig. 4.2 Intraoperative images demonstrating (**a**) the placement of biologic mesh cut in a "C" configuration and anchored to the diaphragm at the esophageal hiatus with sutures; (**b**) the biologic mesh reflected anteriorly to expose the posterior hiatal closure and the right crural relaxing incision; and (**c**) placement of fibrin sealant over the relaxing incision and hiatal closure prior to replacement of the biologic mesh

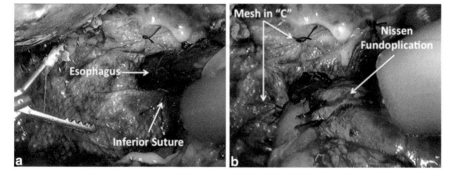

Fig. 4.3 Intraoperative images demonstrating (**a**) biologic mesh reinforcing the hiatus after application of fibrin sealant; (**b**) the final appearance of the esophageal hiatus after placement of mesh, fibrin sealant, and creation of fundoplication

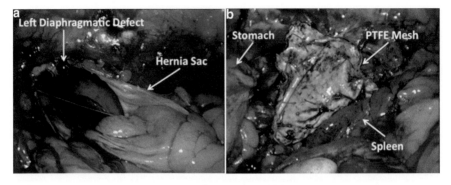

Fig. 4.4 Intraoperative images demonstrating (**a**) iatrogenic hernia of the *left* diaphragm at the site of a previous relaxing incision and (**b**) coverage of the hernia with permanent mesh

matic defect were to develop. Nevertheless, this was not supported by our results, and *we have since changed our practice to patch left-sided incisions with permanent synthetic mesh (Fig. 4.4)*. When doing so, we are careful to secure the mesh in such a way that it does not come in contact with the esophageal muscle.

Reduction in Hiatal Tension Using Pleurotomy and Diaphragmatic Relaxing Incisions

In the same study that identified the anatomic factors that contribute to radial tension at the hiatus (see previous section), Bradley et al. [14] measured the effect of pleurotomy and diaphragmatic relaxing incisions on reducing hiatal tension. Both pleurotomy and diaphragmatic relaxing incisions were associated with a significant reduction in hiatal tension. In six patients who underwent an intentional pleurotomy as the first maneuver to reduce hiatal tension, primary closure of the hiatus was still not possible, and a right diaphragmatic relaxing incision was performed. The addition of a relaxing incision resulted in a 20 % further reduction in hiatal tension and facilitated hiatal closure. Although this study demonstrates relaxing maneuvers objectively reduce hiatal tension to facilitate closure of the difficult hiatus, these authors did not report on any clinical outcomes (e.g., recurrent hiatal hernia) of these patients.

Clinical Effectiveness of Diaphragmatic Relaxing Incisions

Alicuben et al. are the only group to have reported on the clinical outcome of the use of relaxing incisions to facilitate difficult diaphragmatic closure [33]. In their study, 82 patients underwent laparoscopic hiatal hernia repair, and relaxing incisions were performed in 10 (12 %) patients (eight right-sided, one left-sided, and one bilateral). In 69 patients at median follow-up of 5 months postoperatively, 3 (4 %) patients were found to have a recurrent hiatal hernia (all detected on upper endoscopy); only one of these recurrences occurred in a patient who had undergone diaphragmatic relaxing incision.

We recently completed a review of our experience with relaxing incisions to facilitate closure of complex hiatus. We presented this data at the Society of Gastrointestinal and Endoscopic Surgeons 2015 national meeting, and we have submitted it as a peer-reviewed publication. Between 2007 and 2013, we laparoscopicaly repaired 230 primary PEH and 138 recurrent hiatal hernias. Twenty-nine (7.9 %) patients (14 primary PEH and 15 recurrent hiatal hernias) underwent relaxing incision with biologic mesh reinforcement (right $n=22$, left $n=3$, bilaterally $n=1$). We have radiologic follow-up in 146 patients (median follow-up 9 months, range 6–83) with a total of 66 (45 %) recurrent hiatal hernias detected on follow-up esophagram. There was no difference in the rate of recurrence among the three different groups: Primary closure of the hiatus (21/36 [58 %]), primary closure with biologic mesh reinforcement (36/94 [38 %]), and relaxing incision with biologic mesh reinforcement (9/16 [56 %]) ($p=0.428$). Reoperation was needed in four patients. Two patients developed a recurrent hiatal hernia associated with significant dysphagia; one originally underwent primary hiatal closure without mesh and one primary hiatal closure with mesh. Two additional patients presented with symptomatic diaphragmatic hernias through left-sided relaxing incisions that had been covered with biologic mesh. At reoperation, the hernias were each repaired using permanent synthetic mesh. No hernias occurred through right-sided relaxing incisions. There were no gastroesophageal complications associated with use of biologic mesh at the hiatus, and there was no mortality due to any of the operations.

Our resultsdemonstratethree main findings: First, the incidence of recurrent hiatal hernia in patients who undergo hiatal closure with relaxing incisions is similar to patients who undergo primary closure of the hiatus with or without biologic mesh reinforcement. Second, biologic mesh may be safely substituted for synthetic mesh when used to cover a right-sided relaxing incision. Third, permanent synthetic mesh should be used to cover left-sided relaxing incisions, because use of biologic mesh in this capacity is associated with the development of a diaphragmatic hernia.

Gastropexy for the Unclosable Hiatus

In rare situations, the esophageal hiatus is truly un-closable. When faced with this situation, one option is reduction of the stomach into the abdominal cavity and performance of anterior abdominal wall gastropexy. The fixation of the stomach can be performed with sutures and/or tube gastrostomy.

We recently published our experience with laparoscopic anterior abdominal wall-sutured gastropexy for obstructive gastric volvulus [34]. Over a 6-year period, we laparoscopically repaired 357 paraesophageal hernias and performed laparoscopic gastropexy in 11 patients (six with chronic gastric volvulus and five with acute gastric volvulus). A gastropexy was performed in this very select group of patients due to significant cardiopulmonary disease that placed them at a prohibitively

Fig. 4.5 Schematic
demonstrating placement
of sutures (*circles*) and,
when used, gastrostomy
tube (*star*) during anterior
abdominal wall-sutured
gastropexy

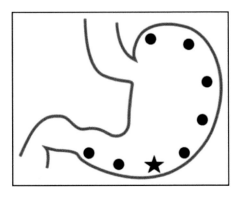

high risk for formal paraesophageal hernia repair. The median age of these patients
was 83 (range 50–92).

During laparoscopic gastropexy, the stomach is reduced as much as reasonably
possible. Then, beginning at the left crus, permanent sutures are placed between the
greater curvature of the stomach and the diaphragm and anterior abdominal wall
(Fig. 4.5). In our experience, a gastrostomy tube was placed in 10 of 11 patients, but
it was only used in one patient. Furthermore, two patients experienced significant
postoperative complications secondary to the gastrostomy tube. Based on this expe-
rience, now we selectively place gastrostomy tubes in patients who we predict will
be unable to tolerate adequate oral nutrition. Although the number of patients was
small and clinical follow-up was limited, no patient has returned with obstructive
symptoms following this modified suture gastropexy technique. Although this study
reviewed patients who underwent gastropexy due to high risk for prolonged surgery,
subsequently we have used this technique in two patients due to an unclosable hiatus with good short-term results, but no long-term follow-up.

Conclusions

Tension-free closure of the esophageal hiatus is a key step to the success of laparoscopic hiatal hernia repair, because hiatal tension is thought to be a contributing
factor to the development of recurrent hiatal hernia. In some patients, primary
tension-free diaphragmatic closure is not possible. The use of permanent mesh to
reinforce the hiatal closure has been fraught with complications, and biologic mesh
reinforcement of the hiatus does not reduce the long-term rate of recurrent hiatal
hernia. Autologous tissue flaps, including the falciform ligament and the left triangular ligament, allow for reinforcement of hiatal closure or bridging of a hiatus that
cannot be closed without the introduction of a foreign body, synthetic or biologic.
Diaphragmatic relaxing incisions and intentional pleurotomy objectively reduce
radial tension at the esophageal hiatus, facilitating primary tension-free closure.

Initial investigations suggest these techniques are safe; however, their long-term clinical effectiveness at reducing recurrent hiatal hernia remains unknown. Major questions remain unanswered concerning these techniques, including which patients will benefit and which technique is preferred. Larger studies with more comprehensive pre- and postoperative symptom evaluation andsystematic long-term radiographic follow-up are needed to answer these questions and assess whether these techniques can reduce recurrent hiatal hernias.

References

1. Oelschlager BK, Pellegrini CA, Hunter JG, Brunt ML, Soper NJ, Sheppard BC, et al. Biologic prosthesis to prevent recurrence after laparoscopic paraesophageal hernia repair: long-term follow-up from a multicenter, prospective, randomized trial. J Am Coll Surg. 2011;213(4):461–8.
2. DeMeester SR. Laparoscopic paraesophageal hernia repair: critical steps and adjunct techniques to minimize recurrence. Surg Laparosc Endosc Percutan Tech. 2013;23(5):429–35.
3. Alicuben ET, Worrell SG, DeMeester SR. Resorbable biosynthetic mesh for crural reinforcement during hiatal hernia repair. Am Surg. 2014;80(10):1030–3.
4. Fortelny RH, Petter-Puchner AH, Glaser KS. Fibrin sealant (Tissucol) for the fixation of hiatal mesh in the repair of giant paraesophageal hernia: a case report. Surg Laparosc Endosc Percutan Tech. 2009;19(3):e91–4.
5. Watson DI, Thompson SK, Devitt PG, Smith L, Woods SD, Aly A, et al. Laparoscopic repair of very large hiatus hernia with sutures versus absorbable mesh versus nonabsorbable mesh: a randomized controlled trial. Ann Surg. 2015;261(2):282–9.
6. De Moor V, Zalcman M, Delhaye M, El Nakadi I. Complications of mesh repair in hiatal surgery: about 3 cases and review of the literature. Surg Laparosc Endosc Percutan Tech. 2012;22(4):e222–5.
7. Pérez Lara FJ, Fernández JD, Quecedo TG, Lafuente FC, Muñoz HO. Mesh extrusion into the esophageal lumen after surgery for a giant hiatal hernia. Am Surg. 2014;80(12):E364–6.
8. Tatum RP, Shalhub S, Oelschlager BK, Pellegrini CA. Complications of PTFE mesh at the diaphragmatic hiatus. J Gastrointest Surg. 2008;12(5):953–7.
9. Wassenaar EB, Mier F, Sinan H, Petersen RP, Martin AV, Pellegrini CA, et al. The safety of biologic mesh for laparoscopic repair of large, complicated hiatal hernia. Surg Endosc. 2012;26(5):1390–6.
10. Stadlhuber RJ, Sherif AE, Mittal SK, Fitzgibbons RJ, Michael Brunt L, Hunter JG, et al. Mesh complications after prosthetic reinforcement of hiatal closure: a 28-case series. Surg Endosc. 2009;23(6):1219–26.
11. Ward KC, Costello KP, Baalman S, Pierce RA, Deeken CR, Frisella MM, et al. Effect of acellular human dermis buttress on laparoscopic hiatal hernia repair. Surg Endosc. 2015;29(8):2291–7.
12. Oelschlager BK, Pellegrini CA, Hunter J, Soper N, Brunt M, Sheppard B, et al. Biologic prosthesis reduces recurrence after laparoscopic paraesophageal hernia repair: a multicenter, prospective, randomized trial. Ann Surg. 2006;244(4):481–90.
13. Van Helsdingen CF. Hiatal herniorrhaphy with posterior gastropexy utilizing the ligamentum teres hepatis. Int Surg. 1968;50(2):128–32.
14. Bradley DD, Louie BE, Farivar AS, Wilshire CL, Baik PU, Aye RW. Assessment and reduction of diaphragmatic tension during hiatal hernia repair. Surg Endosc. 2014;24:1–9.
15. Ponka JL. The relaxing incision in hernia repair. Am J Surg. 1968;115(4):552–7.

16. Petro CC, Como JJ, Yee S, Prabhu AS, Novitsky YW, Rosen MJ. Posterior component separation and transversus abdominis muscle release for complex incisional hernia repair in patients with a history of an open abdomen. J Trauma Acute Care Surg. 2015;78(2):422–9.
17. Horvath KD, Swanstrom LL, Jobe BA. The short esophagus: pathophysiology, incidence, presentation, and treatment in the era of laparoscopic antireflux surgery. Ann Surg. 2000;232(5):630–40.
18. Luketich JD, Grondin SC, Pearson FG. Minimally invasive approaches to acquired shortening of the esophagus: laparoscopic Collis-Nissen gastroplasty. Semin Thorac Cardiovasc Surg. 2000;12(3):173–8.
19. Oelschlager BK, Yamamoto K, Woltman T, Pellegrini C. Vagotomy during hiatal hernia repair: a benign esophageal lengthening procedure. J Gastrointest Surg. 2008;12(7):1155–62.
20. Urbach DR, Khajanchee YS, Glasgow RE, Hansen PD, Swanstrom LL. Preoperative determinants of an esophageal lengthening procedure in laparoscopic antireflux surgery. Surg Endosc. 2001;15(12):1408–12.
21. Lamb PJ, Myers JC, Jamieson GG, Thompson SK, Devitt PG, Watson DI. Long-term outcomes of revisional surgery following laparoscopic fundoplication. Br J Surg. 2009;96(4):391–7.
22. Ringley CD, Bochkarev V, Ahmed SI, Vitamvas ML, Oleynikov D. Laparoscopic hiatal hernia repair with human acellular dermal matrix patch: our initial experience. Am J Surg. 2006;192(6):767–72.
23. Varga G, Cseke L, Kalmár K, Horváth OP. Prevention of recurrence by reinforcement of hiatal closure using ligamentum teres in laparoscopic repair of large hiatal hernias. Surg Endosc. 2004;18(7):1051–3.
24. Varga G, Cseke L, Kalmar K, Horvath OP. Laparoscopic repair of large hiatal hernia with teres ligament: midterm follow-up: a new surgical procedure. Surg Endosc. 2008;22(4):881–4.
25. Laird R, Brody F, Harr JN, Richards NG, Zeddun S. Laparoscopic repair of paraesophageal hernias with a falciform ligament buttress. J Gastrointest Surg. 2015;19(7):1223–8.
26. Park AE, Hoogerboord CM, Sutton E. Use of the falciform ligament flap for closure of the esophageal hiatus in giant paraesophageal hernia. J Gastrointest Surg. 2012;16(7):1417–21.
27. Ghanem O, Doyle C, Sebastian R, Park A. New surgical approach for giant paraesophageal hernia repair: closure of the esophageal hiatus anteriorly using the left triangular ligament. Dig Surg. 2015;32(2):124–8.
28. Monasch S. The relaxing incision in the anterior rectus sheath in the operative treatment of inguinal hernia. Arch Chir Neerl. 1965;17(1):13–21.
29. Pauli EM, Rosen MJ. Open ventral hernia repair with component separation. Surg Clin North Am. 2013;93(5):1111–33.
30. Pauli EM, Wang J, Petro CC, Juza RM, Novitsky YW, Rosen MJ. Posterior component separation with transversus abdominis release successfully addresses recurrent ventral hernias following anterior component separation. Hernia. 2014;19(2):285–91.
31. Huntington T. Laparoscopic mesh repair of the esophageal hiatus. J Am Coll Surg. 1997;184(4):399–400.
32. Greene CL, DeMeester SR, Zehetner J, Worrell SG, Oh DS, Hagen JA. Diaphragmatic relaxing incisions during laparoscopic paraesophageal hernia repair. Surg Endosc. 2013;27(12):4532–8.
33. Alicuben ET, Worrell SG, DeMeester SR. Impact of crural relaxing incisions, Collis gastroplasty, and non–cross-linked human dermal mesh crural reinforcement on early hiatal hernia recurrence rates. J Am Coll Surg. 2014;219(5):988–92.
34. Yates RB, Hinojosa MW, Wright AS, Pellegrini CA, Oelschlager BK. Laparoscopic gastropexy relieves symptoms of obstructed gastric volvulus in highoperative risk patients. Am J Surg. 2015;209(5):875–80.

Chapter 5
Laparoscopic Nissen Fundoplication: Pitfalls and Pearls in Going from Learning Curve to Expert

Nathaniel J. Soper

Rudolf Nissen, in 1956, was the first surgeon to report plicating the fundus of the stomach around the lower esophagus to prevent gastroesophageal reflux. It is said that he thought this operation might work because he had previously excised a distal esophageal ulcer and buttressed the closure with the wrapped fundus. Over the ensuing years, he noted the patient to be free of heartburn. The initial fundoplications for GERD were performed by laparotomy at the University of Basel [1]. Over the ensuing years, a number of variations on the fundoplication were described, and in 1991, Dallemagne reported the first laparoscopic Nissen fundoplication [2]. The application of a minimally invasive approach to the esophageal hiatus simplified the operation, resulted in considerably less perioperative pain and morbidity than its open counterpart, and resulted in an increased application of fundoplication for the treatment of GERD [3]. The basic requirement to be termed a "Nissen fundoplication" is that the upper fundus of the stomach is wrapped 360° around the posterior aspect of the esophagus and fixed in place. Nissen initially reported fully mobilizing the fundus by dividing the short gastric vessels, but several of his disciples subsequently advocated performing a 360° wrap without short gastric vessel division (Rosetti modification) [4]. The more common variation of the Nissen fundoplication was popularized by DeMeester as the "short floppy" fundoplication with full fundic mobilization and a wrap less than 2.5 cm in length [5]. The majority of surgeons now perform the short floppy fundoplication, but many of the specific operative details vary tremendously between different surgical "experts."

It is important for the practicing surgeon to not only understand the essential principles of an effective fundoplication, but also to appreciate the various technical details that differ among experts. As the Nissen fundoplication is a functional, rather than ablative, procedure, these technical principles must be carefully

N.J. Soper, M.D. (✉)
Department of Surgery, Northwestern Memorial Hospital,
251 East Huron Street, Suite 3-105, Galter Pavilion, Chicago, IL 60611, USA
e-mail: nsoper@nm.org

© Springer International Publishing Switzerland 2016   55
R.W. Aye, J.G. Hunter (eds.), *Fundoplication Surgery*,
DOI 10.1007/978-3-319-25094-6_5

followed to result in good long-term functional outcomes. The essential principles for a Nissen fundoplication are as follows:

1. *The esophagus must be protected from injury during dissection, never directly grasped or manipulated with traumatic instruments, and all dissection performed under direct vision.*
2. *The mediastinal esophagus must be mobilized enough so that at least 3 cm of esophagus lies caudad to the hiatus in order to allow for a fundoplication to be performed around the esophagus and below the diaphragm.*
3. *The anterior and posterior vagal trunks must be protected from injury.*
4. *The fundus, rather than any other part of the stomach, must be plicated around the esophagus, rather than around the proximal stomach. The fundus exhibits vagally mediated receptive relaxation, allowing for a lower pressure conduit.*
5. *There must be no tension on the fundoplication, either axial (tending to pull the repair up through the hiatus into the mediastinum) or rotational (pulling the fundus counter-clockwise back to the left, creating a twist of the lower esophagus).*
6. *The right and left surgical crura should be approximated without tension such that they touch the walls of the empty esophagus at the conclusion of the case.*

The following text will describe the basic technical details of the laparoscopic Nissen fundoplication and describe pitfalls often encountered, together with potential "pearls" which may facilitate surgical evolution to achieve expertise.

Patient Positioning and Equipment

The patient must be carefully positioned to protect both the patient and the surgeon—the patient from neuromuscular injury while under general anesthesia and the surgeon from undue muscular fatigue and poor ergonomics. The patient's legs are abducted, preferably on flat padded boards, which allows the knees to be extended and minimizes the potential for lower extremity neurovascular traction injury as is more likely to occur when using stirrups. The surgeon will stand between the patient's legs facing directly forward during the operation. Video monitors are placed at the head of the table to allow ergonomically neutral visualization by the surgeon and assistants. During the operation, the patient will be positioned in the steep reverse Trendelenburg position. This positioning fulfills two functions: the omentum and abdominal viscera fall away from the diaphragm by gravity, and the patient's torso is brought closer to the surgeon, thereby allowing the surgeon to stand fully erect. The patient must be secured in position to avoid sliding inferiorly. We prefer a vacuum bean bag mattress that provides general support around the patient's sides and perineum to prevent intraoperative movement. The right arm is tucked inside the bean bag to allow the liver retractor to be fixed to the right side of the table.

Performance of the laparoscopic Nissen is facilitated by the use of specific instrumentation. An angled laparoscope, either 30° or 45°, allows for adjustable and alternative views of the operative field, facilitating adequate visualization of the retrogastric and retroesophageal regions, as well as high into the mediastinum. An adequate atraumatic liver retractor is necessary to allow the left lateral section of the liver to be elevated for prolonged periods without capsular injury. This liver retractor is held in a self-retaining device to maximize hiatal exposure and minimize fatigue of the assistant as well as potential liver damage from repetitive repositioning. We use a number of atraumatic grasping and dissecting instruments, including ones with Babcock type and DeBakey type tips. Appropriate instrumentation for achieving hemostasis and dividing tissues bloodlessly should be used: we primarily use an ultrasonic coagulating shears, but others use bipolar electrosurgical devices—this is per surgeon preference. Importantly, a flexible gastroscope should be present in the room to allow intraluminal evaluation of the esophagus and stomach as necessary.

Annotated Steps of the Operation

Abdominal Access and Port Placement

Although either an open or closed technique may be used to access the peritoneal cavity, we prefer to use the Veress needle in the vast majority of cases. Port positioning depends on the personnel available. We prefer to have a dedicated camera holder sitting to the left side of the patient, able to freely change the viewing angle on a second by second basis. We put the initial camera port 12 cm inferior to the xiphoid in the left mid-rectus such that it is off midline, but lateral to the ligamentum teres and medial to the inferior epigastric vessels. In general, the esophageal hiatus is located dorsal to the xiphoid process. Port positioning should allow the midpoint of instruments to be located at the level of the abdominal wall (fulcrum) to maximize their range of motion during tissue manipulation and to establish a one to one ratio between external hand movements and internal instrument tip translations. As most laparoscopic instruments are 30–35 cm in length, we therefore position the laparoscopic ports in an arc 10–15 cm inferior to the xiphoid process and costal arch (Fig. 5.1).

The esophagus generally enters the abdomen in a slightly right to left orientation and the falciform ligament and liver limit the distance to the right of midline the port for the surgeon's lcft hand can be placed; this is why we generally place the laparoscope port to the left of the midline. The preferred position is almost always superior to the umbilicus—*in general, a periumbilical port site is too far inferior on the abdominal wall for operations at and above the esophageal hiatus.* The surgeon's right hand port is generally placed 10 cm from the xiphoid and in a subcostal position and the surgeon's left hand port position is just inferior and to the right of the xiphoid process beneath the right subcostal margin. The left upper quadrant port is 10 mm diameter to allow insertion of an SH needle. This port positioning allows the laparoscope to be located between the operating hands with the surgeon working straight ahead and avoiding mirror imaging. This also allows maximization of visual cues for accurately perceiving three-dimensional relationships. We place the liver

Fig. 5.1
Port placement

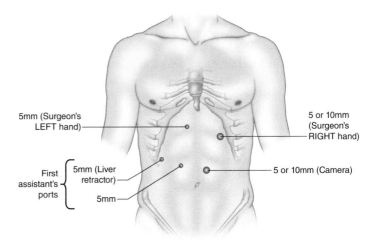

5mm (Surgeon's LEFT hand)

5 or 10mm (Surgeon's RIGHT hand)

First assistant's ports { 5mm (Liver retractor) 5mm

5 or 10mm (Camera)

retractor port in the right abdomen 15 cm from the xiphoid in a subcostal position. The assistant's port is placed in the right mid-rectus region approximately midway between the liver retractor port and the camera port. We generally place the port for the surgeon's left hand instruments last, after the liver retractor has been inserted and secured in position. This is because the precise location of this port depends to a large extent on the size and location of the liver in its retracted position. We use a Veress needle to "sound out" potential sites on the abdominal wall for this port before the incision is made and the final trocar and sheath are inserted.

If a dedicated camera operator is not present, the surgical assistant will hold the camera in the left hand while manipulating an instrument with the right hand. Under these circumstances, the assistant's working port is placed 15 cm from the xiphoid in the left subcostal region. Other surgeons prefer the laparoscopic camera port to be placed in a midline position or at the umbilicus. These alternative port positions are valid, but we generally insert the ports as noted above for the reasons given.

Pitfalls and Pearls

1. *Long and difficult laparoscopic fundoplications may result in musculoskeletal pain of the surgeon: During advanced laparoscopic procedures, the surgeon must optimize the positioning of the ports, the patient, and the video monitors to be as ergonomically favorable as possible.* If the table is too high, the shoulders and supraspinatus muscles may bear the brunt. When the monitors are positioned too high, the cervical muscles can be strained. In general, the monitors should be placed at a level below the surgeon's eyes. During the primary portion of the dissection, the surgeon must continually strive to maintain the elbows as close to the body as possible to avoid strain on the rotator cuffs. Finally, it may be worth-

while to take "mini breaks" throughout the procedure, as when a surgeon is focused on the laparoscopic image, it can be easy to lock into a position, resulting in joint pain. Brief periods of stretching and change of positions can improve one's musculoskeletal comfort throughout the operation and potentially prolong the career of the surgeon.

Hiatal Dissection

The assistant grasps the anterior wall of the stomach and pulls it inferiorly and to the left, placing traction on the gastrohepatic ligament. This is divided with an energy source, generally also dividing the hepatic branch of the vagus nerve and any small aberrant left hepatic arteries with impunity. The gastrohepatic ligament is divided up to the level of the right crus of the diaphragm. The assistant then grasps the epiphrenic fat pad, which is uniquely situated to be a major point of traction during the operation, and retracts caudad. The ultrasonic shears is used to divide the anterior phrenoesophageal membrane transversely, being careful to keep this dissection superficial to avoid injury to the underlying esophagus and anterior vagal trunk. The superior part of the fundus is then pulled inferiorly and to the left to allow division of the gastrophrenic ligament, thereby freeing the cardia of the stomach in preparation for esophageal mobilization. *During the remainder of the dissection, the surgeon should strive to leave peritoneum and/or endoabdominal fascia on the crura to allow a more robust primary suture approximation.*

We start the esophageal dissection just medial to the base of the right crus of the diaphragm by insinuating a blunt-tipped instrument and widely opening its jaws in a vertical orientation. This initiates a plane between the esophagus and the right crus; the left hand instrument pushes the crus to the patient's right, while the right hand instrument gradually and gently sweeps the esophagus and periesophageal tissue to the left to bluntly mobilize the right side of the distal esophagus. *Attempts should be made to identify the posterior vagus nerve quickly and to use that structure as marking the posterolateral dissection plane;* the posterior vagus trunk is swept anterior and to the left alongside of the esophageal wall to mobilize the esophagus from the seven o'clock position to the ten o'clock position. *Keep in mind that the posterior vagus sometimes traverses the hiatus considerably posterior to the esophagus and can be injured if not identified early.* With mild esophagitis, this dissection is usually quick, performed bluntly and bloodlessly, and without the use of energy. In patients with significant periesophageal inflammation, however, the plane may be much more difficult to develop and often the right pleura can extend across the midline or even be intimately adherent to the lateral wall of the esophagus. This mobilization continues in a cephalad direction as far as possible and then back distally to the level of the right crus. Dissection then continues around the anterior aspect of the esophagus with the surgeon's left hand retracting the anterior arch and pericardium anteriorly, while gently teasing the esophagus away from the pericardium. The surgeon's left hand then slides around to the left side to elevate the left crus away from the esophageal wall and the periesophageal tissue is swept away from the crus to develop a plane to the left of the esophagus. The anterior vagus nerve should be seen at this time and be used as a dissection plane, swiping the anterior vagus back toward the esophagus. The initial dissection of the mediastinum is therefore completed, freeing the esophagus from the pleura, aorta, and lateral crural attachments. The anterior and posterior vagus nerves are clearly identified and maintained alongside the esophagus to avoid subsequent injury.

Pitfalls and Pearls

1. Dissection of a large hernia sac can be problematic: *In the presence of a large hiatal hernia, the hernia sac itself must be reduced and the stomach will come with it back to the abdominal cavity.* The pneumoperitoneum pressure will exert cephalad tension on the hernia sac similar to a fully deployed spinnaker on a sail boat. To deal with the hernia sac quickly and effectively, the right crus is grasped and elevated anteriorly with the left hand, while the assistant reaches high and pulls the hernia sac (just medial to the crus) in a caudad direction and to the left to place it on tension. The ultrasonic shears is then used to divide the hernia sac approximately 1 cm medial to the crural muscle in an effort to retain some of the peritoneum and endoabdominal fascia on the crus. After the sac is divided, one enters the plane between the sac and the mediastinal structures. Using blunt dissection, the hernia sac is then swept medially and inferiorly away from the crus and from the right pleura. The assistant retracts the hernia sac vigorously, while the surgeon bluntly develops the plane between the sac and the mediastinal structures. *When the correct plane is entered, it is avascular and the majority of the dissection is performed bluntly without need for an energy source.* The dissection is carried around the anterior two thirds of the hiatal orifice, progressively dividing the hernia sac and reducing it bluntly toward the abdomen. With large hernias, there is both an anterior hernia sac and a posterior hernia sac, the latter corresponding to the lesser sac. After dividing the short gastric vessels, the posterior sac can likewise be divided medial to the crural orifice and the remaining sac reduced. *The anterior and posterior vagal nerves should be identified and used as planes for dissection, maintaining the vagi on the esophagus and dissecting other structures away from them.* Likewise, the aorta posteriorly serves as a good dissection plane, dividing any sac anterior to this and trying to avoid dissecting to the left side of the aorta as this increases the risk of damage to the left pleura.
2. Inadvertent injury to the pleura may result in hypotension and elevated airway pressure: A laceration or tear of the pleura is relatively common when repairing large hiatal hernias. This occurs in approximately one third of operations for paraesophageal hiatal hernias, whereas the incidence is well less than 10 % in standard Nissen fundoplications without a large hernia component. When a pleural tear occurs, there is a capnothorax of pure CO_2 under a controlled pressure and without damage to the underlying lung parenchyma. *The anesthetist should be informed of the pleural injury. Occasionally, patients will become hypoten-*

*sive transiently; this virtually always resolves with decreasing the pneumoperi-
toneum pressure and increasing positive pressure ventilation.* Rarely, and in the
presence of scarring such as a re-operation, there can be a ball valve effect with
development of a true tension pneumothorax. The response to this event would
be to enlarge the hole in the pleura to create a common cavity and to reduce the
intrapleural pressure. In our experience of more than 2000 laparoscopic hiatal
operations, a chest tube has only been placed once intra-operatively and this was
early in our series. When a capnothorax has occurred, our routine at the end of
the operation is to place a suction catheter into the mediastinum through the
hiatal closure and aspirate during exsufflation of the pneumoperitoneum while
the anesthesiologist administers vital capacity breaths. *Unless the patient has
difficulty with oxygenation or ventilation, a routine chest X-ray is not performed
postoperatively, as it may lead to inappropriate interventions.*

3. After reducing the hernia sac, it may have considerable bulk at the EGJ, interfering
   with visualization and tissue manipulation: Particularly in patients with significant
   intra-abdominal adiposity, the hernia sac itself may be sizeable and contain much
   redundant tissue that may be difficult to retract for exposure. We will usually
   debride as much of the hernia sac as possible, particularly those areas that appear
   to be devascularized. The danger when excising the hernia sac is that one may
   injure the vagus nerves or the actual wall of the stomach or esophagus. We generally start this debridement by grasping the hernia sac toward the right side of the
   esophagus, elevating it and retracting caudad and to the patient's right. *This generally places the anterior vagus nerve on tension, rendering its location and course
   obvious.* The hernia sac to the left of the esophagus is elevated and the harmonic
   shears are used to divide the sac to the left of the anterior vagus nerve posteriorly
   to the EGJ and then to the left of the esophagus. Likewise, the posterior sac can
   also be removed in similar fashion, being careful to visualize the posterior vagus.
   It is better to leave some of the sac in place than risk damage to the underlying
   EGJ. Often the tissue mass is significant and not easily removed through the
   laparoscopic ports. We tear the tissue into smaller pieces to be removed quickly
   through the 11 mm port site in the left subcostal region.

Mobilization of the Fundus

The gastric fundus is then mobilized to allow a subsequent tension-free wrap. The
lateral border of the fundus is grasped and retracted anteriorly and to the right, while
the gastrosplenic ligament is grasped and retracted ventrally and to the left. A point
is selected on the greater curvature 10–15 cm inferior to the angle of His, but cephalad to the most proximal gastroepiploic vessels. With adequate tension on the tissue,
the ultrasonic shears divide a short gastric vessel close to the stomach wall, with the
aim being to enter the lesser sac as quickly as possible. Once the lesser sac is entered,
the lateral border of the greater curvature of the stomach is aligned with the visual
axis of the laparoscope. The energy device is then used to simply march up the

greater curve, sequentially dividing the short gastric vessels and all other attachments that would otherwise tether the stomach. As the cephalad portion of the fundus is reached, the dissection plane joins the previously created plane at the infero-medial edge of the left crus.

Complete mobilization of the greater curvature of the fundus enhances visualization of the high retrogastric space, facilitating division of the gastropancreatic ligaments and the posterior gastric vessels. The short gastric vessels should be divided close to the insertion on the stomach wall to limit the amount of extraneous material left in situ that will need to be dealt with during the fundoplication. Furthermore, the sites of insertion of these vessels pinpoint the lateral border of the fundus, marking the most mobile part of the stomach, which will later be used for the fundoplication. After completing this fundic mobilization, the retroesophageal space is visualized from the anatomic left side. The medial border of the left surgical crus of the diaphragm is dissected back to its junction with the right crus, joining the plane previously begun from the right side. A window is thereby created under direct vision posterior to the EGJ and anterior to both crura.

Once this window is created, many surgeons place a Penrose drain around the esophagus for inferior traction on the EGJ. This is a useful maneuver and should be encouraged if traction is difficult to achieve by other means, but may be somewhat time-consuming. We generally skip this step and instead use traction on the epiphrenic fat pad or the fundus itself. Following the posterior mobilization, a grasper is placed through the retroesophageal window from right to left which then grasps the apex of the fundus and pulls it back through the window and to the right side of the esophagus. With caudad traction placed on the wrapped fundus itself, the EGJ and distal esophagus can be brought further into the abdominal cavity.

Once the fundus has been pulled to the right side, it is checked for rotational tension and torsion. *To assess rotational tension, the wrapped fundus is released and observed. If it recoils back around the esophagus to the left, there is tension that must be eliminated by mobilizing additional fundic attachments. To check for a twist or entrapment of the wrapped fundus in the posterior window, a "shoe shine" maneuver is performed (Fig. 5.2). The fundus is retracted back and forth to make sure that it slides easily and is not twisted or overly redundant.*

Prior to closing the crura and constructing the fundoplication, one must assure adequate intra-abdominal esophageal length. Traction on the EGJ is released and the length of intra-abdominal esophagus is measured. This should be greater than 2.5–3 cm to allow placement of the fundoplication within the abdomen. If adequate intra-abdominal length is not evident, additional esophageal mobilization or an esophageal lengthening procedure (see Chap. 3) needs to be performed.

Pitfalls and Pearls

1. Difficulty exposing and dissecting the lateral aspect of the fundus; in a patient with visceral adiposity, a bulky omentum may make this dissection problematic: Assure that the reverse Trendelenburg position has been maximized. Sometimes

Fig. 5.2 The "shoeshine"
maneuver

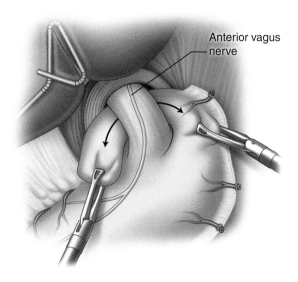

Anterior vagus
nerve

simply placing an unfolded 4×4 sponge in the dissection plane can impede the omental encroachment. At other times, we have found it helpful to place a long length of suture into the abdomen, perform a wide-based figure of eight stitch on the leading edge of the omentum, and then feed both of the suture tails back out of the abdomen alongside the left upper quadrant port site and clamp the suture tails at the level of the skin. The most crucial part of this dissection is to gain access to the lesser sac such that the posterior wall of the stomach can be clearly visualized. The surgeon and assistant then align the lateral aspect of the fundus with the horizontal visual axis of the laparoscope. Often, at the site of the highest short gastric vessel, the fundus and spleen are in very close proximity. Great care must be taken to dissect this space without tearing the splenic capsule. Certainly, err on the side of damaging the gastric wall instead of the spleen. A typical pitfall by trainees is that the gastric wall is pushed forcefully in a cephalad fashion against the diaphragm, allowing no room for dissection. Rather, insinuate the tips of an atraumatic instrument held in the surgeon's left hand caudad to the edge of the gastric wall, open the jaws horizontally, *and elevate the fundus anteriorly while turning the jaws slightly in a clockwise manner to retract the fundus in a ventral direction, away from the diaphragm and underlying spleen.*

2. Difficulty visualizing the retroesophageal hiatus: Following full mobilization of the fundus, it should be possible to roll the fundus in a counter-clockwise direction to the patient's right and exert ventral tension. Sometimes if an oral gastric tube has been placed by the anesthesiologist, this tube may stiffen the tissue-limiting retraction and should be removed after gastric decompression. An angled, rather than a 0° scope, markedly facilitates visualization of this area.

3. *The intra-abdominal esophageal length seems to be inadequate: It is easy to optimistically assess the length of intra-abdominal esophagus as being more than it is in actuality, particularly if even a small amount of caudad traction is being exerted at the EGJ.* All tension on the stomach should be released and then the abdominal esophageal length is measured. We generally use an atraumatic grasper whose jaws, when fully open, measure a distance of 2.5 cm. We also tend to decrease the intra-abdominal pressure slightly during this maneuver such that the diaphragm is not artificially tented in a cephalad direction. In cases with severe inflammation or Barrett's esophagus, it may be difficult to conclusively identify the EGJ laparoscopically. *Under these conditions, intraoperative flexible endoscopy should be performed to identify the squamocolumnar junction and/or the top of the gastric folds.* Should additional esophageal length be needed, traction to the EGJ must be exerted in a caudad fashion either using a Penrose drain or by blunt traction on the epiphrenic fat pad. *It should be possible to mobilize the esophagus up to the inferior pulmonary vein unless one's port positions are too low on the abdominal wall.* Again, using the vagal trunks to mark the dissection plane, a combination of blunt and sharp dissection is performed as high as possible and then the esophageal length is remeasured. Should this still be less than 2.5 cm, a lengthening procedure will be needed (Chap. 3). Over time, and with more objective assessment of intra-abdominal length, our practice has been to perform increasing numbers of esophageal-lengthening procedures.

Crural Closure

The crura are then re-approximated, beginning posterior to the esophagus. As the diaphragmatic hiatus, when viewed from below, is shaped as an inverted teardrop, the posterior pillars are generally closer together and can be more easily closed without tension. Esophageal dilators are not placed prior to crural closure, because the stiffness of the intubated esophagus inhibits access to the retroesophageal space. Traction on the EGJ is maintained ventrally and to the patient's left to expose the crura, either using an atraumatic grasper on the wrapped fundus or with a Penrose drain sling (Fig. 5.3). We generally use interrupted large gauge, braided polyester sutures on an SH needle for this purpose. If a surgeon uses monofilament sutures for this closure, it is appropriate to use pledgets to reinforce the crural sutures. The intra-abdominal crural fascia/peritoneum is incorporated in the sutures rather than simply re-approximating the muscle body alone. Closure begins posteriorly near the crural junction and then proceeds anteriorly towards the esophagus, until the crura lightly touch the walls of the empty esophagus. We generally also place at least one anterior suture to stimulate some scarring in this area, as most recurrent hiatal hernias occur anterior to the esophagus. *Once the crural closure is completed, it should be possible to pass a 5-mm instrument between the esophagus and the crura.* In patients with very large hiatal hernias, it may be impossible to close the crura without undue tension. Management of the difficult diaphragmatic closure is covered in Chap. 4.

Fig. 5.3 Closure of the crura posterior to the esophagus

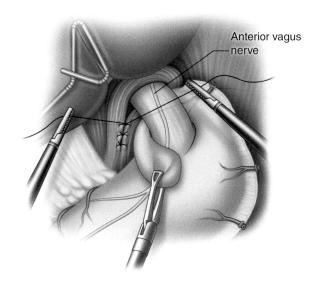

Anterior vagus nerve

Pitfalls and Pearls

1. Difficulty in placing crural sutures: Adequate ventral tension must be maintained at the EGJ to expose the base of the crura; this visualization is markedly improved by the use of an angled laparoscope. We place the first suture approximately 1 cm ventral to the junction of the surgical crura. *My mandate to trainees is to take large bites of tissue, "everything but aorta."* We prefer using an SH needle to be able to reliably know the depth and arc of the needle tip. It is often helpful during closure of the crura to decrease the intra-abdominal pneumoperitoneum pressure and thereby diminish the tension on the diaphragm. *When it becomes difficult to securely fashion intracorporeal knots due to tension, I become concerned that the closure is under too much tension and that additional measures should be used. If there is undue tension, we tend to perform a relaxing incision to the right of the right crus and then patch the resulting defect with a long-term resorbable mesh. Due to the rounded contour of the ventral aspect of the hiatus, it is easy to place sutures that overly tighten the crural closure anteriorly. After placing each anterior stitch, the suture ends should be crossed to assess the degree of tissue approximation before tying the knot. The balance between sutures placed in the crura anterior and posterior to the esophagus depends ultimately on the course of the esophagus as it traverses the diaphragm; angulation should be minimized.*

Fundoplication

After more than two decades of performing laparoscopic fundoplications, we still advocate placing an in-dwelling bougie dilator during creation of the wrap. This step is probably not imperative as long as the surgeon has adequate experience with laparoscopic suturing, understands the three-dimensional relationships, and avoids excessively narrowing the EGJ. Depending on the size of the patient and whether or not strictures have been present, we serially pass a 50 French and then a 60 French Maloney dilator and suture the fundoplication with the 60 French dilator in place. After the dilator has been placed, the two sides of the fundus are abutted around the distal esophagus to ascertain whether a tension-free wrap may be achieved. The lateral edge of the fundus to the left of the esophagus is sutured to the leading edge of the wrapped fundus to the right of the esophagus. In general, three 2-0 gauge, braided polyester sutures on SH needles are used, taking deep seromuscular suture bites in the fundus to the left and right of the esophagus. The sutures are placed approximately 1 cm apart, thereby achieving a length of fundoplication between 2 and 2.5 cm. At least one of the sutures incorporates the anterior muscularis of the esophagus to the right of the anterior vagus nerve. The first suture opposes fundus to fundus without incorporating the esophageal wall, as there may be tension on the tissue while approximating the two leafs of the fundoplication. After this first suture is tied, the location and orientation of the wrap are checked and the fundoplication may be slid up or down the esophagus in order to position its caudad edge just proximal to the EGJ. Great care must be taken during knotting of the sutures, particularly the one incorporating the esophageal wall, to prevent anterior traction, which could cause a tear of the esophageal or gastric wall. We generally tie these sutures using intracorporeal knotting techniques.

   After completing the suturing, the dilator is removed and the wrap is checked for its degree of laxity by passing a 5-mm diameter instrument between the left side of the wrap and the esophagus. *We measure the length of the wrap to ensure it is less than 2.5 cm and make sure that it is situated around the esophagus rather than more inferiorly on the proximal stomach (Fig. 5.4).* The suggested orientation of the wrap (the point on the esophagus at which the two sides of the fundus are joined) varies in different centers. Some surgeons advocate that this junction be placed at the right lateral position of the esophagus, at nine o'clock, presumably to minimize lateral traction. We tend to place the sutures to the right of the anterior midline of the esophageal wall at the eleven o'clock position with the esophageal suture placed just to the right of the anterior vagus nerve.

Pitfalls and Pearls

1. Concern about esophageal perforation while placing the dilator: In more than two decades of performing laparoscopic esophageal surgery, we have only experienced one esophageal perforation during placement of the Maloney dilators. In that case, the dilator had "expired" and was very stiff. Thus, one should be

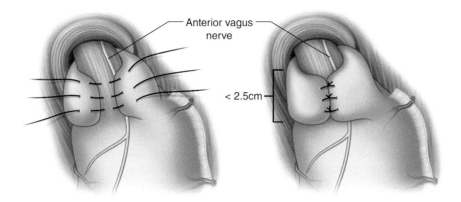

Anterior vagus
nerve

< 2.5cm

Fig. 5.4 Final appearance of the fundoplication

sure that the dilators are appropriately malleable. Some surgeons advocate scrub-
bing out and placing the dilators themselves. I believe this is time-consuming
and generally trust my anesthesia colleagues to place dilators under direct laparoscopic visualization. *We maintain good communication between the individual
inserting the dilator and the surgical team. During dilator placement, the EGJ is
maintained in a non-angulated position by the surgeon and assistant and the
anesthesiologist calls out the distance of the tip from the incisors while slowly
passing the dilator well into the stomach along the lessor curve.* It is likely that
the most common cause of dilator perforation is due to the tip of the dilator
bending back on itself and then causing a tear on the anterior wall of the EGJ due
to the increased tension of the doubled dilator.

2. *Difficulty placing the fundoplication sutures: There is a fine balance between the
   wrap being too tight, leading to dysphagia, or too loose, leading to a herniation
   of redundant fundus or recurrent reflux.* The shoe shine maneuver should assure
   that there is no redundancy of the fundus as it passes posterior to the esophagus.
   This can more clearly be seen while exerting inferior traction on the Penrose
   drain or on the epiphrenic fat pad to create a furrow along the left side of the
   esophagus and to clearly visualize the arc of the fundus as it "hugs" the wall of
   the esophagus in its posterior passage.

   *Choosing the site on the fundus to place sutures can be confusing initially. We
   use the lateral border of the fundus, indicated by the stumps of the short gastric
   vessels, as the anatomic landmark for suturing. Sutures are placed between the
   anterior aspect of the fundus to the left of the esophagus and the posterior aspect
   of the wrapped fundus (medial to the vessels) to the right of the esophagus. This
   orientation can be clarified early in a surgeon's experience by placing a marking
   suture on the fundus (prior to wrapping) ~2 cm posterior to the vessels and
   ~3–5 cm distal to the angle of His. This suture can be grasped by an instrument
   passed from right to left behind the esophagus and used as the "lead point" of
   the wrap.*

We tend to place the most caudad suture in the fundoplication first so that the wrap can be positioned just proximal to the EGJ. If the proximal suture is placed first, the wrap may end cephalad to the EGJ, thereby exposing the distal esophageal mucosa to acid. These fundoplication sutures should be seromuscular in nature and not full thickness, as there have been reports of gastric ulcers developing at the site of intramucosal sutures. If there is any doubt regarding the appearance of the fundoplication, intraoperative endoscopy should be performed. On retroflexed view, the typical "stacked coins" appearance should be present, indicating a normal Nissen fundoplication. Many variations of fundoplication fixation have been described, including "crown" sutures, sutures between the wrap and crura, etc. We generally do not fix the wrap to the diaphragm given the fact that the EGJ moves in a different plane during swallowing than the diaphragm moves during breathing, sneezing, etc.

Completing the Operation

After removing the dilator, the esophageal hiatus is once again assessed. Occasionally, it will become apparent that there is still a gap in the crural closure and additional sutures may be added. The liver retractor is removed and the undersurface of the liver is examined for capsular tears or bleeding. The upper abdomen is aspirated and checked for hemostasis. The ports are then removed under direct vision. For any port larger than 5 mm in diameter that was created using a cutting trocar and is located below the costal margin, one should strongly consider closing the fascia with heavy gauge suture. The abdomen is exsufflated, the ports are removed, and each incision is infiltrated with long acting local anesthetic.

Postoperative management includes routine use of antinauseants and intravenous anti-inflammatory drugs to minimize the need for narcotics, as vomiting or retching in the early postoperative period is associated with a significantly elevated recurrence rate. We no longer perform routine postoperative contrast studies. However, if the patient vomits or retches in the early postoperative period or experiences undue chest pain, a water-soluble contrast swallow study is performed. If the retching led to an acute herniation, the patient should immediately be taken back to the operating room for re-repair. Significant postoperative complications directly related to the fundoplication can occur, but are rare (less than 1 %). Gastric perforations due to seromuscular tears caused by a traumatic instrument or by an inadvertent thermal injury may occur requiring a reoperation. Esophageal leaks due to direct injury may also occur, which may require a thoracotomy. With complex hiatal dissections, particularly in the face of significant periesophageal inflammation, pleural effusions may develop. It is also possible to damage the thoracic duct with the posterior hiatal dissection. During an operation, should chyle appear in the field, deep figure of eight sutures should be placed in the posterior mediastinum to occlude the thoracic duct. If a chylothorax is diagnosed postoperatively, it should be managed conservatively or approached by interventional radiology percutaneously placing coils in the thoracic duct at the hiatus.

Our routine is to allow the patient sips of clear liquids the evening of the operation. We maintain all patients in the hospital overnight and then assess their ability to tolerate a full liquid diet the morning following surgery. Should the patient have no problem with oral liquids, a dental mechanical soft diet is offered at lunch time and the patient is discharged early in the afternoon. We generally maintain patients on the soft diet for 2–4 weeks postoperatively depending on the degree of initial dysphagia the patient experiences. In general, in the presence of normal esophageal motility, the incidence of ongoing dysphagia should be less than 5 %.

References

1. Liebermann-Meffert D. Rudolf Nissen (1896–1981)—perspective. J Gastrointest Surg. 2010;14(Supp 1):S58–61.
2. Dallemagne B, Weerts JM, Jehaes C, Markiewicz S, Lombard R. Laparoscopic Nissen fundoplication: preliminary report. Surg Laparosc Endosc. 1991;1:138–43.
3. Wang YR, Dempsey DT, Richter JE. Trends and perioperative outcomes of inpatient antireflux surgery in the U.S., 1993–2006. Dis Esophagus. 2011;24:215–23.
4. Rossetti ME, Liebermann-Meffert D. Nissen-Rosetti fundoplication (open procedure). In: Baker RJ, Fischer JE, editors. Mastery of surgery. Philadelphia: Lippincott, Williams & Wilkins; 2001. p. 764–77. Chap. 60.
5. DeMeester TR, Johnson LE, Kent AH. Evaluation of current operation for the prevention of gastroesophageal reflux. Ann Surg. 1974;180:511–8.

Chapter 6
Alternatives to Nissen Fundoplication: The Hill Repair and the Nissen-Hill Hybrid

Heather Warren and Ralph W. Aye

Introduction

In 1967, Lucas D. Hill introduced the Hill Repair to the American Surgical Association, and it transformed the field of antireflux surgery [1]. The principles behind the Hill repair were derived from detailed anatomical dissections and incorporated the regular use of preoperative and intraoperative esophageal manometry and pH testing. The science and objective measures behind the Hill repair not only facilitated the creation of a highly effective and durable antireflux operation, but also set standards in an emerging field that continue to be utilized in present day [2, 3]. *Incorporating the knowledge and technical aspects of the repair into one's repertoire enhances the understanding of the function and anatomy of both the gastroesophageal junction (GEJ) and its modification by antireflux procedures and broadens the surgical options available for both straightforward and complex surgical repairs.*

Advantages of the Hill Repair

1. *Proven efficacy and durability* [2, 4]
2. *Accurately reproduces normal anatomy, with inferior fixation of the gastroesophageal junction (GEJ) and complete reconstruction of the antireflux barrier without reliance on a fundoplication, thus reducing herniation and wrap slippage and enabling use following partial gastrectomy or gastric bypass* [5, 6].

H. Warren, M.D.
Department of Thoracic Surgery, Swedish Medical Center, Seattle, WA, USA

R.W. Aye, M.D., F.A.C.S. (✉)
Department of Thoracic and Foregut Surgery, Swedish Cancer Institute,
Swedish Medical Center, 1101 Madison, Suite 900, Seattle, WA 98104, USA
e-mail: ralph.aye@swedish.org

© Springer International Publishing Switzerland 2016
R.W. Aye, J.G. Hunter (eds.), *Fundoplication Surgery*,
DOI 10.1007/978-3-319-25094-6_6

3. *Esophageal lengthening procedure generally not required, even in instances of short esophagus* [7].
4. *Intraoperative manometric control over the final lower esophageal sphincter (LES) pressure, allowing for an individualized tailored surgical repair. Suitable for patient with ineffective esophageal motility and a very low incidence of long-term dysphagia* [8].
5. *Maintenance of the short gastric vessels and associated low incidence of postoperative gas bloat* [5].

Principles of Repair

The Hill repair incorporates three important anatomical concepts: (1) the intra-abdominal posterior fixation of the GEJ; (2) the central role of the collar sling musculature of the LES in the proper reconstruction of the GEJ; and (3) the importance of the gastroesophageal valve (GEV) for the competence of the antireflux barrier, while adhering to traditional tenets of antireflux surgery, including closure of the crura, configuring an intra-abdominal segment of distal esophagus, and reestablishing total/intra-abdominal length and pressure of the LES.

The anatomical reconstruction of the GEJ is accomplished through the Hill repair sutures, which anchor the anterior and posterior aspects of the LES collar sling musculature to the preaortic fascia just superior to the celiac trunk. A thorough understanding of the LES anatomy facilitates proper placement of the Hill sutures. As previously delineated by Liebermann-Meffert, the clasp fibers of the lesser curvature on the LES interdigitate with the collar sling musculature of the oblique gastric muscle layer, the latter of which forms a horseshoe arching over the anterior, posterior, and greater curvature (angle of His) aspects of the GEJ (Fig. 6.1) [9]. Four successively placed Hill sutures through the sling fibers allow for progressive downward tension on the sling fibers and accentuation of the angle of His. Intraoperative manometry is utilized to assess appropriate tension of the Hill sutures and allows for an individualized tailoring of the valve and antireflux barrier [10].

Hill Repair Technique

A complete list of the equipment required for a laparoscopic Hill antireflux procedure can be found in Table 6.1.

Manometry Catheter and Bougie Dilator Placement

The manometric equipment is prepared prior to initiation of the operation. The manometry catheter is a water-perfused, single-use eight channel catheter, with four pressure ports at 0 cm from the tip, and subsequent ports at 5-cm intervals.

Fig. 6.1 Diagrammatic illustration of the collar sling musculature

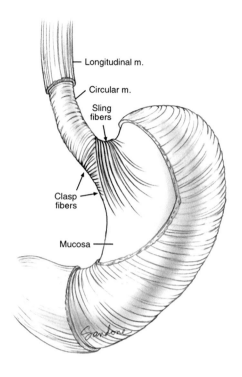

Table 6.1 Equipment used in the Hill repair

Instrument	Manufacturer	Catalog number
Manometry catheter	Sierra scientific instruments	9012P1222
Bougie dilator	Cook medical, Winston Salem NC	
Wingman Scope Holder	Stryker endoscopy	240-240-000
Nathanson liver retractor	Cook medical	G26912, C-NLRS-1001
		G26913, C-NLRS-1002
Self-retaining table mount	Thompson surgical	90011B
Ti-knot: device	LSI solutions	030404
Ti-knot: knots	LSI solutions	030510
48 in. 0 ethibond	Ethicon endosurgery multipack	22970D8684

The catheter is placed through a clear 44–48 Fr dilator with the distal pressure port 10 cm beyond the tapered tip of the dilator and secured with tape at the proximal end. The bougie and attached catheter is then passed through the esophagus to 30 cm at the beginning of the case by the surgeon or an experienced anesthesiologist, taking care that the manometric catheter remains properly oriented and is not folded upon itself. The distal channel is connected to a transducer and anesthesia monitor—at pulmonary artery catheter settings for greatest sensitivity—or to a dedicated esophageal manometry system.

Patient Positioning and Port Placement

Our standard positioning is low dorsal lithotomy with both arms out at 90°. The surgeon stands between the legs, the assistant on the patient's left, and the camera operator or robotic arm for camera fixation on the right. Five trocars are used for the operation. It is noteworthy that a 10–11 mm assistant port is placed just below the left costal margin in the mid-clavicular line, or more medially when the costal margin is narrow. This requires placement of the surgeons' right-hand work port more inferiorly than would be typical for a Nissen repair (Fig. 6.2a), but the assistant port location facilitates management of the Hill sutures (Fig. 6.2b). A sixth optional port for downward traction of lesser curvature fat may be added in the left lower quadrant to gain better exposure to the preaortic fascia; this exposure is critical to placement of the preaortic sutures and may be particularly helpful with obese patients. The left lobe of the liver is elevated with a 5-mm Nathanson retractor and fixed to a self-retaining table mounted system.

Hiatal Dissection and Closure

Dissection is performed with ultrasonic shears. Care is taken to dissect along the superior aspect of the phrenoesophageal fat pad (Hill's phrenoesophageal bundle) and bring it down with the dissection, keeping it attached to the GEJ. Following dissection, the anterior and posterior fat pad/bundles are trimmed as necessary to eliminate hernia sac and redundancy, while avoiding the lesser curvature and the vagus nerves. *The short gastric vessels are not routinely taken, but it is essential with a Hill*

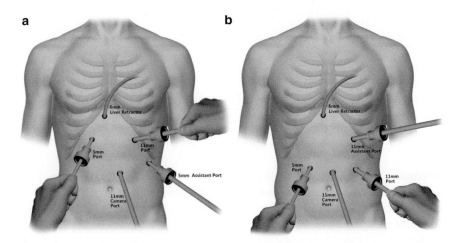

Fig. 6.2 (**a**) Trochar placement for the laparoscopic Nissen and Nissen-Hill hybrid repair. (**b**) Trochar placement for the laparoscopic Hill repair

repair to free the entire posterior fundus by opening the lesser sac from left gastric artery to GEJ. This is accomplished from the lesser curvature aspect and facilitated with critical exposure provided by the assistant, who lifts the posterior phrenoesophageal tissue immediately posterior to the posterior vagus nerve. The location of the celiac trunk should be roughly identified (though not dissected) and the preaortic fascia and overlying diaphragmatic muscle should be exposed down to the level of the celiac axis. (The preaortic fascia is a dense connective tissue layer that lies deep to the inferior fusion of the right and left crura and extends inferiorly to the celiac axis, where its inferior edge forms the median arcuate ligament.) Dissection is continued into the mediastinum to obtain adequate length of intra-abdominal esophagus. A Penrose drain is not routinely utilized, as it would be in the way of subsequent suture placement. Following dissection, the hiatus is closed posteriorly with 0-braided non-absorbable suture using an extracorporeal knot pusher or the Ti-Knot device. *For larger hernias, some of the hiatal repair may need to be completed anteriorly, since too much angulation of the esophagus may be created from excessive posterior closure and subsequent posterior fixation of the GEJ to the preaortic fascia.*

Hill Sutures: Anatomical Landmarks

The Hill sutures are placed through the collar sling musculature of the GEJ (see Fig. 6.1). This lies immediately beneath the phrenoesophageal ligament (Hill's phrenoesophageal bundles), commencing just to the patient's left and anterior to the anterior vagus nerve, extending over the angle of His and ending just to the patient's right and posterior to the posterior vagus nerve. Thus, the vagus nerves are important landmarks and must be identified. The anterior vagus nerve is found under tension by pulling down on the lesser curvature tissue. The posterior vagus nerve is found by lifting the posterior fat pad upward and to the patient's right, as it consistently lies in the groove between the fundus and esophagus created by this maneuver. It is usually necessary to trim part of the anterior and posterior esophageal fat pads to delineate the appropriate anatomy.

Hill Sutures: Placement

Following hiatal closure, four Hill sutures of multicolored 48 in. 0-Ethibond are placed and left untied and clamped externally. *This is the most critical part of the repair, and exact placement is important (Fig. 6.3).* The first two sutures are introduced through the surgeon's right-hand working port, while the third and fourth are introduced through the assistant port in the left upper quadrant. *There are three separate and distinct bites of tissue with each suture, the first being placement through the anterior bundle/collar sling musculature from inferior to superior; the second being placement through the posterior bundle/collar sling musculature from*

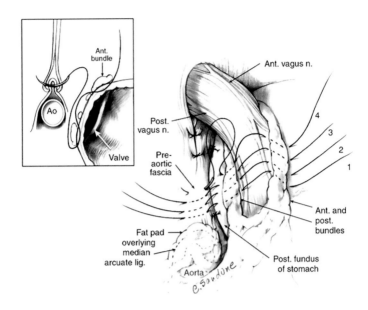

Fig. 6.3 Illustration of the Hill sutures

superior to inferior; and the third being transverse placement through the inferior aspect of the preaortic fascia. Placement of the posterior bundle sutures may be aided by preliminarily fixing the superior aspect of the posterior fundus to the left crus and left aspect of the preaortic fascia with 1–2 sutures.

Anterior Bundle: The first bite of the first suture is placed immediately to the patient's left of the anterior vagus nerve. Grasping the bundle with the left hand and maneuvering the tissue over the needle facilitates this placement. This bite must go deeply enough to grab the collar sling musculature, and as previously discussed, it is usually necessary to trim away part of the anterior fat pad to expose this anatomy (Fig. 6.4).

Posterior Bundle: The second bite of the same suture is placement through the posterior bundle. The assistant exposes the posterior vagus nerve by grasping the lesser curvature tissue between the vagus nerves and retracting it anteriorly and to the left. The surgeon grasps and manipulates the posterior bundle with the left hand. Beginning just posterior to the posterior vagus, the suture is passed through the bundle in a superior to inferior direction, including the underlying collar sling musculature. To do this successfully, the needle will frequently need to be perpendicular to the tissue at the time of entry (Fig. 6.5).

Preaortic Fascia: The final bite is transverse placement through the preaortic fascia. The assistant retracts the GEJ to the left and inferiorly for exposure. The suture is passed through the preaortic tissue inferiorly, immediately superior to the fatty tissue overlying the celiac axis. *The location of this suture determines the final length of intra-abdominal esophagus, so it is important to be sufficiently inferior.*

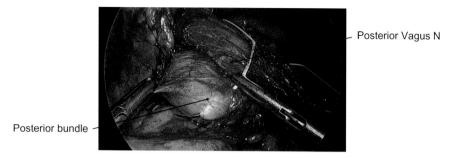

Fig. 6.4 First Hill suture, first bite: intraoperative view

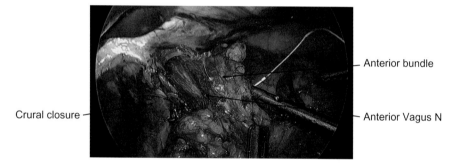

Fig. 6.5 First Hill suture, second bite: intraoperative view

The aorta lies 5–10 mm deep and may be avoided by lifting the tissue upward with a grasper and *driving the needle transversely from left to right, rather than posteriorly (Fig. 6.6)*. Finally, the suture is then retracted through the working port, taking care to brace the suture internally with a grasper to avoid excess tissue trauma. It is then clamped externally with a hemostat (Fig. 6.7).

This same process is repeated with three more sutures; the second suture also going through the surgeon's right hand work port, while the third and fourth sutures are introduced and withdrawn through the left upper quadrant assistant port. Each suture advances 2–3 mm further up the two bundles (e.g., in the direction of the angle of His) and the preaortic fascia. With excessive advancement, the repair will be too snug, whereas with inadequate advancement the repair may be too loose. The uppermost suture should enter the anterior bundle at approximately the left lateral border of the esophagus. It should enter the posterior bundle at its upper extent without going behind the esophagus. Colors should alternate to aid in identification and prevention of tangling. *Care should be given to the angle of entry of the sutures through the ports, to also prevent crossing.* Three-eighths inch Teflon pledgets may be added to either end of the sutures; it has been our standard to add pledgets to the second and fourth sutures.

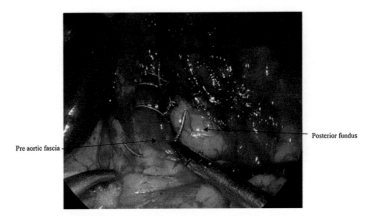

Fig. 6.6 First Hill suture, third bite: intraoperative view

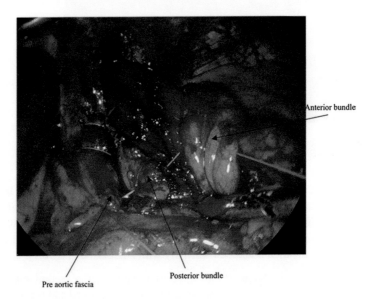

Fig. 6.7 First Hill suture, completed but not tied: intraoperative view

Hill Sutures: Fixation and Manometric Measurements

With all repair sutures placed but not tied, the 48 Fr dilator/manometry catheter is carefully advanced and positioned across the GEJ, and the top 2 sutures, i.e., those through the left assistant port, are tied sequentially with a single half-hitch and clamped internally just above the knots with needle holders. The left hand instrument clamps the most superior suture, while the right-hand instrument clamps the second inferior suture. *These two sutures are highest on the collar sling musculature and will therefore have the greatest impact on lower esophageal sphincter pressure.*

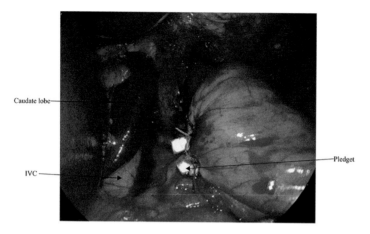

Fig. 6.8 Completed Hill repair: intraoperative view

Manometric measurements are taken by withdrawing the dilator/catheter system until the pressure port is 5 cm below the repair. A relative baseline intragastric pressure of zero should be established by raising or lowering the transducer, and fixing it at that point, the catheter is then slowly withdrawn at a rate of 1 cm/s. This should be done more slowly if an arterial monitor is used, especially during crossing of the high-pressure zone, in order to capture the highest peak. The ideal pressure is 30–40 mmHg. The first increase in pressure encountered during pull-through is the repair, whereas an additional spike representing the diaphragm may be seen just proximal to this.

The manometric pressure of the GEJ may then be adjusted by tightening or loosening the Hill sutures as needed. If the pressure is clearly too low, an additional superior suture may be placed as deemed appropriate. When satisfactory pressure has been obtained, the dilator is again positioned across the GEJ and all sutures are extracorporally tied at the established tension before taking a final manometric reading. Figure 6.8 shows the completed Hill repair.

The Hill repair may be performed over a 40–45 Fr bougie without the use of intraoperative manometrics, as many of Hill's former students have done. In our experience, intraoperative manometrics has altered the operation approximately 30 % of the time [10].

Completion of the Repair

The anterior hiatus is often reinforced with one or two sutures to prevent further attenuation and as a preferred alternative to excess posterior closure. Mesh may be used at the discretion of the surgeon, but excess posterior bulk should be avoided. The fundus is sutured to the anterior rim of the hiatus along both right and left crura, to prevent herniation and accentuate the valve.

Postoperative Care

Postoperative care is standard. Nasogastric suction is not routinely utilized. The patient is kept on full liquids for 2 weeks, and then advanced slowly to a normal diet by 6 weeks.

Results of the Hill Repair

The Hill repair is highly effective and durable. The durability of the Hill repair was shown in a large multi-institution study of 1184 patients with long-term follow-up (2–25 years, mean follow-up of 10 years), demonstrating a 93 % long-term clinical success rate and only a 1.9 % reoperation rate [2]. The Hill repair has been successfully translated into laparoscopic technique, with over 2500 laparoscopic repairs having been performed. Clinical results have been nearly identical to the open repair [3]. The effectiveness and safety of the Hill repair has also been demonstrated for patients with diminished esophageal peristalsis [8], and for those with para-esophageal hernia and short esophagus, without the need for an esophageal lengthening procedure [7].

The Hill repair has also been compared to the standard Nissen fundoplication. In a recent multi-institution randomized controlled trial comparing the laparoscopic Nissen and Hill repairs, the Hill was equivalent to the Nissen in every parameter of clinical success and repair failure, including symptomatic and physiologic control of reflux, except that, in contrast to the Nissen repair it did not raise lower esophageal sphincter pressure significantly above baseline. This may be an advantage in cases of ineffective esophageal motility. There was also a trend toward less gas bloating [3]. The results of this updated study supersede the only other randomized comparison of the two operations, done in the 1970s [11] in which the Nissen was deemed superior; however, the sample size and description of the Hill technique in that study raises concern about the standardization and quality of the Hill repair that was performed.

A failure of the Hill repair is clinically apparent with the return of reflux symptoms in the setting of positive pH testing, with or without evidence of a recurrent hiatal hernia on an upper gastrointestinal series (Figs. 6.9 and 6.10). The initial failure is believed to result from loosening and attenuation of the anterior bundle repair sutures, as a result of radial forces, which decreases the fixation and strength of the GEJ. As with any reoperative procedure, the technical difficulty is greater than that of the primary repair, principally as a result of the increased difficulty of dissection [12]. Careful attention to dissection of the posterior bundle sutures and fundus from the preaortic fascia is required. Barring any contraindications, such as significant esophageal dysmotility, we have managed recurrent disease with conversion of the Hill Repair to the Nissen-Hill Hybrid Repair.

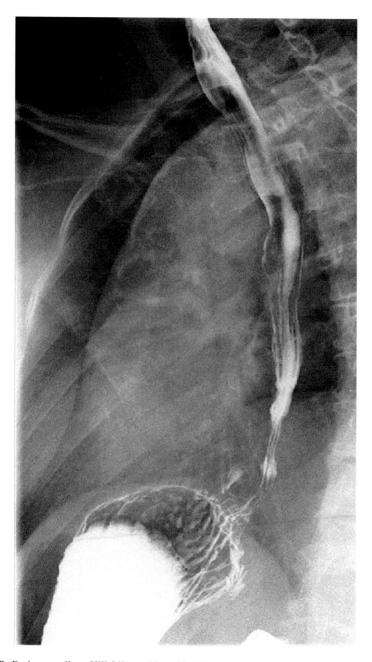

Fig. 6.9 Barium swallow: Hill failure without hiatal hernia recurrence

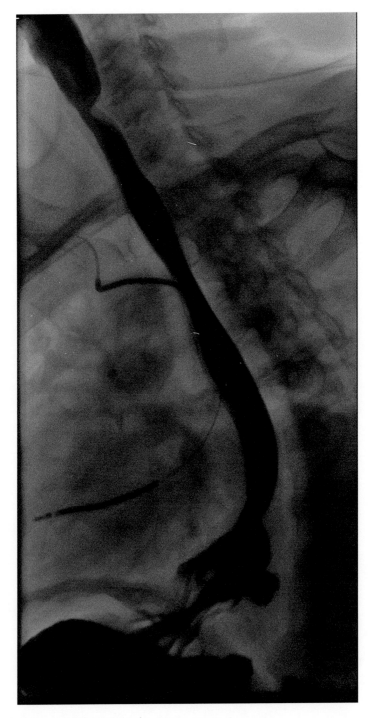

Fig. 6.10 Barium swallow: Hill failure with hiatal hernia recurrence

The Nissen-Hill Hybrid Repair

The Nissen-Hill hybrid has become our preferred repair for reoperations, parae-sophageal hernias, and in cases of short esophagus. As previously discussed, the most common failure of the Hill repair is from loosening and attenuation of the anterior bundle sutures, with herniation of the GEJ being relatively uncommon [3]. Contrarily, the most common failure of the Nissen fundoplication is mediastinal herniation of the wrap; the second most common failure is a slipped Nissen, result-ing from cephalad herniation of the GEJ and cardia through the wrap, with the wrap remaining intra-abdominal [3, 13]. Both of these failures reflect inadequate fixation of the GEJ within the abdomen. In a recent randomized trial comparing 46 Nissen fundoplications to 56 Hill repairs, there were two reoperations in the Nissen group, both for mediastinal herniation of the wrap; and there were two reoperations in the Hill group, both for loosening of the repair [3].

The Nissen-Hill hybrid repair incorporates the structural features of both repairs, offsetting the weakness of one repair with the integrity of the other. Two Hill sutures securely anchor the GEJ within the abdomen to maintain axial integrity, while a full 360° Nissen wrap maintains radial integrity. It is not simply an anchored Nissen wrap, in that it is the GEJ, rather than the wrap, which is anchored, resulting in complementary merger of the two repairs.

Nissen-Hill Hybrid Technique

Positioning and dissection are as described for the Hill repair, except that the port placement is as it is for a Nissen repair, with the surgeon's right-hand work port higher beneath the left costal margin and the 5 mm assistant port placed left lateral, just below the costal margin (see Fig. 6.2a). The dissection is similar except that the short gastric vessels are routinely taken and a Penrose drain is placed around the GEJ for downward traction during mediastinal dissection and construction of the Nissen wrap. The gastroesophageal fat pad and associated hernia sac are routinely removed except along the lesser curvature, taking care to protect both vagus nerves. The hiatus is closed posteriorly with 0-braided non-absorbable suture.

Following hiatal closure, *there are four components to the Nissen-Hill hybrid repair:*

Nissen Configuration

A marking suture is placed on the posterior fundus by traveling 6 cm below the GE junction along the greater curvature and one third of the distance from greater to lesser curvature. A mirror-image mark is made on the anterior fundus with a marking pen. The posterior fundus is brought behind the esophagus and a "shoe-shine" maneuver is then performed to ensure full mobility of the fundus and a 1:1 relationship between anterior and posterior fundus. No fundoplication sutures are placed at this time.

Placement of Hill Sutures

The two lower of the four standard Hill sutures are then placed through the collar sling musculature and preaortic fascia as previously described (Fig. 6.1) [5]. The ends of each suture are brought out through the trocar, clipped together, and returned into the abdomen and placed inferiorly and laterally out of the field until the Nissen is completed.

Modified Hybrid Repair

In elderly patients or those with poor esophageal motility, Hill suture bites through the anterior collar sling may be omitted, using only bites through the posterior collar sling and the preaortic fascia. This still provides competent posterior intra-abdominal fixation of the GE junction, but without the aggressiveness of the anterior collar sling sutures.

Nissen Construction

The Nissen repair is then completed in a standardized fashion [14, 15] over a 58 Fr dilator utilizing a horizontal mattress 2-0 double-armed prolene suture with double-mounted 5/8″ Teflon pledgets on either side, suturing anterior to posterior fundus and incorporating the wall of the esophagus along its lesser curvature aspect (9:00 position) (Fig. 6.11). The sutures are tied using a Ti-Knot device. Two additional fundus-to-fundus sutures are then placed and tied, 5 mm above and 5 mm below the horizontal mattress suture, to create a 2–2.5 cm "floppy" Nissen wrap (Fig. 6.12).

Completion of the Hill Sutures and EGD

With the dilator in place, the Hill sutures are retrieved in reverse order, redundant tissue along the lesser curvature is retracted inferiorly, and the sutures are tied down with the Tie-knot. Intraoperative manometry is not done as the repair is performed over a large dilator. The laxity of the anterior hiatus is assessed before and after removing the dilator and is typically reinforced and/or further closed with one or

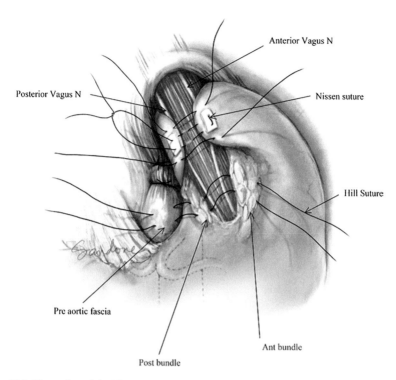

Fig. 6.11 Illustration of the Nissen-Hill hybrid sutures in place (untied)

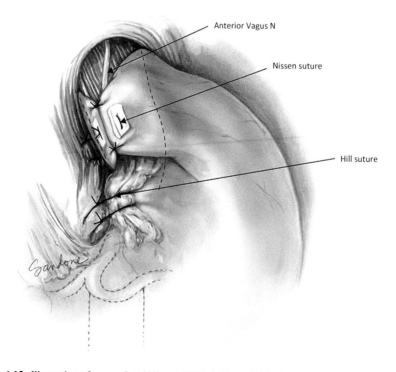

Fig. 6.12 Illustration of a completed Nissen-Hill hybrid repair (tied)

more sutures to prevent subsequent widening and herniation. Biologic absorbable mesh is used routinely in cases of para-esophageal hernia. This should be low-profile material so as not to create excess bulk behind the esophagus. The corresponding intraoperative pictures of the Hybrid repair, with the Nissen already in place, and placement of mesh toward the end can be seen in Figs. 6.13, 6.14, and 6.15.

We routinely perform flexible upper endoscopy to assess calibration of the repair and the valve configuration. This is a helpful tool to aid the surgeon in refining technique and will occasionally prevent a disastrous outcome.

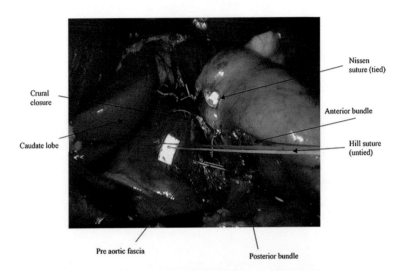

Crural closure

Caudate lobe

Nissen suture (tied)

Anterior bundle

Hill suture (untied)

Pre aortic fascia

Posterior bundle

Fig. 6.13 Nissen wrap completed, hybrid sutures in place: intraoperative view

Fig. 6.14 Completed hybrid repair: intraoperative view

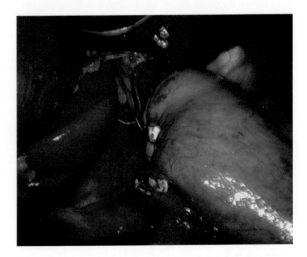

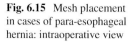

Fig. 6.15 Mesh placement in cases of para-esophageal hernia: intraoperative view

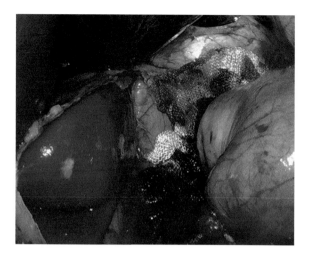

Results of the Hybrid Repair

With short-term follow-up in over 150 hybrid repairs, the results continue to exceed our initial expectations. After an initial feasibility and safety trial on patients with para-esophageal hernia and Barrett's metaplasia [16], the procedure has now been extended to patients with uncomplicated reflux. Gratifyingly, there has been no noticeable increase in complications or short to mid-term side effects, and the recurrence rate has been lower than predicted with traditional repair. In the first 50 patients with para-esophageal hernia undergoing hybrid repair, there was only one clinical recurrence at 13-month follow-up; there were three small asymptomatic fundic herniations with the GE junction intact and no reflux on pH testing; only two patients had resumed antisecretory medication, and preoperative symptoms were controlled in 98 %. There were significant improvements in all parameters of quality of life metrics, including dysphagia [17]. Similar success has been achieved in a smaller group of patients with Barrett's metaplasia.

A recent mid-term cohort analysis of 153 patients who underwent Hybrid, Nissen, or Hill repair for uncomplicated GERD demonstrated an equivalent improvement in quality of life between the three repairs, but significantly reduced dysphagia rate and a trend toward reduced recurrences in those who had a Hybrid repair compared to a standard Nissen or Hill repair [18].

Summary

The Hill repair is at least equivalent in short-term clinical outcomes to the Nissen fundoplication in the surgical management of uncomplicated gastroesophageal reflux, and it may have advantages in the management of short esophagus and ineffective esophageal motility. In addition, as it is based on different anatomic and functional concepts than the Nissen, it gives additional insight into the multi-modality and critical aspects of a successful antireflux operation.

The open repair has been shown to be highly durable with up to 25-year follow-up, and the operation has been successfully translated into a laparoscopic approach, with clinical results that match the open approach. Its technical performance is well within the scope of any qualified esophageal surgeon, and the technical details of manometric calibration and precise suture placement have been standardized and simplified.

The Nissen-Hill hybrid repair incorporates features of each of the individual repairs and acts in a synergistic manner, offsetting the weakness of one with the advantages of the other. Like the Hill repair, it is also particularly useful in cases of short esophagus, as it anchors the GE junction intra-abdominally and obviates the need for an esophageal lengthening procedure. Short- and mid-term results suggest that this approach may be superior to either the Nissen or the Hill in cases of para-esophageal hernia or short esophagus, without an increase in side effects or complications.

References

1. Hill LD. An effective operation for hiatal hernia: an eight year appraisal. Ann Surg. 1967;166(4):681–92.
2. Aye RW, et al. The Hill antireflux repair at 5 institutions over 25 years. Am J Surg. 2011;201(5):599–604.
3. Aye RW, et al. A randomized multi institution comparison of the laparoscopic Nissen and Hill repairs. Ann Thorac Surg. 2012;94(3):951–8.
4. Low DE, et al. Fifteen- to twenty-year results after the Hill antireflux operation. J Thorac Cardiovasc Surg. 1989;98(3):444–9. discussion 449–50.
5. Aye R. The Hill procedure for gastroesophageal reflux [AU1]. 1st ed. Philadelphia: Harcourt Health Sciences; 2001.
6. Aye R, Gupta A. Antireflux surgery: the Hill antireflux operations repair and its variants. New York: Springer; 2014.
7. Jobe BA, et al. Laparoscopic management of giant type III hiatal hernia and short esophagus. Objective follow-up at three years. J Gastrointest Surg. 2002;6(2):181–8. discussion 188.
8. Aye RW, Mazza DE, Hill LD. Laparoscopic Hill repair in patients with abnormal motility. Am J Surg. 1997;173(5):379–82.
9. Korn O, et al. Gastroesophageal sphincter: a model. Dis Esophagus. 1997;10(2):105–9.
10. Schneider A, Aye R. Impact of intraoperative manometry on the Hill repair. Abstract presented at North Pacific Surgical Association, 14–15 Nov 2014. 2014.
11. Demeester TR, Johnson LF, Kent AH. Evaluation of current operations for the prevention of gastroesophageal reflux. Ann Surg. 1974;180(4):511–25.
12. Pennathur A, et al. Minimally invasive redo antireflux surgery: lessons learned. Ann Thorac Surg. 2010;89(6):S2174–9.
13. Horgan S, et al. Failed antireflux surgery: what have we learned from reoperations? Arch Surg. 1999;134(8):809–15. discussion 815–7.
14. DeMeester TR, Bonavina L, Albertucci M. Nissen fundoplication for gastroesophageal reflux disease. Evaluation of primary repair in 100 consecutive patients. Ann Surg. 1986; 204(1):9–20.

15. Attwood SE, et al. Standardization of surgical technique in antireflux surgery: the LOTUS trial experience. World J Surg. 2008;32(6):995–8.
16. Qureshi AP, et al. The laparoscopic Nissen-Hill hybrid: pilot study or a combined antireflux procedure. Surg Endosc. 2013;27(6):1945–52.
17. Aye RW, et al. Laparoscopic Nissen-Hill hybrid: a promising solution for Type III paraesophageal hernia. Abstract Poster presentation at Digestive Disease Week, 20 May, 2013. 2013.
18. Schneider AM et al. Does the Nissen-Hill hybrid repair reduce recurrence rates for uncomplicated GERD? Abstract Poster presentation at Society of American Gastrointestinal and Endoscopic Surgeons 16–17 Apr 2015. 2015.

Chapter 7
Laparoscopic Toupet Fundoplication

David Gotley

Introduction

The individual choice of fundoplication operation remains as controversial now as it did during the working life of Andre Toupet. Not only is there controversy about the extent of fundoplication (Nissen, Toupet, 180° and 90° fundoplication), but also trans-abdominal vs. transthoracic fundoplication and other technical aspects regarding wrap fixation and closure of the hiatus. We will see in this chapter that over time there may be little difference in the clinical results between the above fundoplications, so outcomes will depend upon the technical skills applied by the operating surgeon in constructing the fundoplication in the first place. Poorly constructed fundoplication risks early failure, and revision fundoplication is technically complex surgery. The contemporary requirements of antireflux surgery are that the operation is safe, effective in controlling reflux, has limited side effects, and is durable for the long term. These may seem self-evident, but we should keep all these aims in mind in the era of evolving reflux management, and we should also note that we do not have the ideal operation that fulfils all of these requirements perfectly. It is of immense importance that care and attention are applied to the technical aspects of every fundoplication in order to achieve the best outcomes.

D. Gotley, M.B.B.S., M.D., F.R.A.C.S. (✉)
Princess Alexandra and Mater Private Hospitals, University of Queensland, Brisbane, QLD 4102, Australia

Department of Surgery, Princess Alexandra Hospital, University of Queensland, Ipswich Rd, Brisbane, QLD 4102, Australia
e-mail: d.gotley@uq.edu.au

© Springer International Publishing Switzerland 2016
R.W. Aye, J.G. Hunter (eds.), *Fundoplication Surgery*,
DOI 10.1007/978-3-319-25094-6_7

Historical Aspects

André Toupet was a Parisian surgeon who proposed a partial fundoplication in 1963 that aimed to obviate the post-operative dysphagia seen in 10 % of patients after the full fundoplication of Nissen [1]. He also proposed that the diaphragmatic hiatus not be closed in cases of hiatus hernia, believing that the dilated hiatus was secondary to proximal movement of the gastric cardia into the chest. He believed that satisfactory reduction and careful gastropexy to the hiatal pillars would result in the muscle tone returning to the hiatus, and the dilated hiatus would duly retain its normal size.

His operation as presented to the French Academy of Surgery is published in English in the Annals of Surgery [2]. The principles of the operation involved mobilisation of the abdominal esophagus, mobilisation of the fundus from the diaphragm and posteriorly, but not with division of short gastric vessels. The posterior aspect of the fundus was then brought behind the esophagus to establish the right side of the wrap. This was done by using interrupted sutures between the stomach and the right distal margin of the esophagus, followed by a right posterior gastropexy to the right crus of the diaphragm, again with interrupted sutures. Similarly, a left-sided gastropexy was created between the stomach and the left crus, followed by a line of sutures attaching the gastric fundus to the left distal esophagus. The proximal sutures on each side of the wrap incorporated the diaphragm as well as the stomach and esophagus. The wrap was a posterior hemi (180°) fundoplication. It was initially poorly received, due largely to having only 4 patients with short-term follow-up to present. However, the operation remains popular in Europe and Australia today as it is felt to reduce the risk of dysphagia and gassy side effects and to minimise the risk of post-operative long-term dysphagia in cases where patients have reduced peristaltic activity in the esophagus. These claims will be critically evaluated in this Chapter.

What is a Toupet Fundoplication Today?

Today the term Toupet Fundoplication is generally used for any posterior fundoplication that is less than 360°, with arguably the most common variant being a posterior 270° fundoplication. The circumference of the Toupet wrap is therefore not a prescribed amount in contemporary operations, and it could be varied according to whether a reduced risk of dysphagia or gassy retention is desired, usually between 180° and 270°.

Division of the short gastric vessels is often undertaken in contemporary Toupet operations. The advantage of this is to use the whole of the gastric fundus for the fundoplication, which reduces possible tension on the wrap. On the other hand, it may actually increase gas-bloat side effects [3].

It is now established that closing an open hiatus reduces hernia recurrence rates and therefore reduces recurrent reflux [4]. Toupet's fundoplication not only fixed the wrap to the esophagus by interrupted sutures, but also to the right and left hiatal pillars in similar fashion. While some do not fix the wrap to the hiatal pillars today, it is our view that fixation of the wrap in this way serves to limit trans-hiatal migration and therefore reduces the risk of recurrence.

Why Do Fundoplications Fail?

In thinking about improving the outcomes from fundoplication, it is logical to try to understand why fundoplications fail. In our experience of posterior fundoplications, whether the Nissen or the Toupet, when they do fail it is usually by the same mechanism [5]. We found that the wrap begins to prolapse or herniate through the hiatal ring, and it first occurs posteriorly at the left posterolateral position. The hiatal ring is found to be enlarged, though the posterior previously placed hiatal repair sutures remain present and intact. This implies that the enlargement is at the more anterior part of the hiatal ring. Over time, as the posterior herniation progresses, it distorts the wrap facilitating reflux, and as the wrap moves further into the hiatus it becomes detached anteriorly and is sometimes then pulled apart. It is often assumed that failure is a result of suture dislodgement or sutures cutting out of the tissues, but in our experience of several hundred re-operations we have never found this to be the case. The hiatal laxity is therefore most likely due to enlargement of the hiatus over time, perhaps through abdominal pressure effects, but which does not necessarily occur in all patients after primary fundoplication. Possible precipitating factors as reported by patients may be progressive weight gain, or an extended bout of retching or vomiting, or even sudden straining or lifting, but the initial triggers may be unknown. However, the pattern of disruption is usually the same.

So with this in mind, we should make efforts to reduce the risk factors above. These might include advice about controlling weight and avoiding sudden straining where possible and providing patients with rapid-acting sublingual anti-emetics to use in the case of vomiting. Securing the fundoplication to the hiatal pillars, especially posteriorly, is something we consider important. Such manoeuvres do not appear to increase the prevalence of referred diaphragmatic pain, as is sometimes claimed.

Surgical Technique

Patient Positioning

The operation may be undertaken with the patient supine on the operating table or supine with legs in the lithotomy (or "French") position (usually in padded, moulded leg supports), with reverse Trendelenburg. The advantage of the former is the ease of the patient set-up, but the disadvantage is that the surgeon stands at the patient's side and to access the hiatus the surgeon will need to stand with tilt at the pelvis, which for some causes backache. The lithotomy position allows the surgeon, placed between the legs, to adopt a "face-on" stance toward the operative field, standing symmetrically, equally weighted on both feet. *It makes sense that positive ergonomics and surgeon comfort while operating have longer-term benefits.* The assistant can sit on the left hand side of the patient to hold the camera. Sequential pneumatic calf compression, anti-thrombotic stockings, and fractionated heparin are used for venous thromboembolic prophylaxis.

Fig. 7.1 Laparoscopic
port placement sites

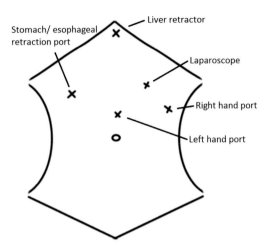

Ports and Placement

With the availability of high definition 5-mm laparoscopes, there is no longer any
need for 10–12 mm ports in fundoplication surgery. Optical entry is safe and avoids
cut-downs which increase tissue trauma. We use 5–7 mm ports, which leave little or
no post-operative pain, allowing early mobilisation, minimal analgesia use, and
confer a low risk of wound infection and port-site herniation.

Port placement is a matter of preference and will depend on the surgical approach
to the hiatus. In our case, since we divide short gastric vessels and dissect the hiatus
and lower esophagus from a left hiatal approach first, the laparoscopic port is placed
in the left upper quadrant in the mid-clavicular line, 5 cm below the costal margin
(Fig. 7.1). We recommend use of a 25–30° laparoscope, which gives better views
lateral to and behind the esophagus than a 0° laparoscope. Operating ports are then
placed on the left side of the abdomen, and in the midline above the umbilicus as
shown. A port for liver retraction is placed in the sub-xiphisternal position. A right
upper quadrant port can be used for retraction of the stomach or the esophagus using
an esophageal sling, as required.

Suturing is facilitated by passing a standard needle down the 7 mm port (Applied
Medical™), after securing the needle point between the jaws of the needle holder in
such a way as to enable the needle to move freely through the port. We usually
employ a pre-formed slip knot.

Omental Retraction

A gathering retraction suture of omentum that overlies the upper greater curve and
spleen, in combination with a soft bowel clamp on the upper greater curve of the
stomach, provides excellent access to the short gastric vessels. This suture can be
withdrawn through the left lateral port, which retracts the attached omentum

inferiorly and laterally from the operative field, and the port is removed and replaced so that suture lies outside the port in the incision. As many of these sutures can be placed as is considered necessary and are especially useful in the obese patient or in cases of a large hiatal hernia.

Liver Retraction

This can be undertaken with either the Nathanson retractor (Cook Group Inc, Bloomington, IN) or a simple ratcheted toothed grasper onto the diaphragm above the right pillar of the diaphragmatic hiatus if the left lobe of the liver is small. The incision/port for this is placed just below the xiphisternum.

Dissection

The dissection is carried out beginning with division of the short gastric vessels, then to mobilisation of the esophagus at the hiatus. Vessel division is undertaken with either harmonic scalpel or bipolar diathermy. *Sometimes the upper short gastric vessels are very short at the superior aspect of the spleen, and easier access can be achieved by approaching the vessels both inferiorly and superiorly by dividing the peritoneal reflection from the gastric fundus to the diaphragm first, and then the peritoneum overlying the vessels. This has the effect of lengthening the exposed vessels for easier division.*

The next step is mobilisation of the esophagus at the hiatus. When mobilising the esophagus on the left lateral side, the phreno-esophageal ligament should be incised 2–3 mm lateral to its insertion into the esophagus, which is usually indicated by a white condensation of the ligament (the "white line"). This avoids inappropriate dissection into the esophageal muscle and readily opens up the lower mediastinal space (Fig. 7.2). The left side and posterior aspect of the esophagus can be easily

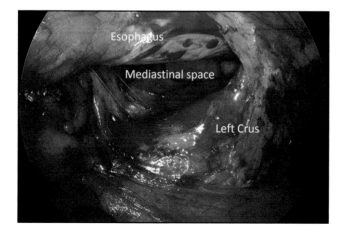

Fig. 7.2 Hiatal dissection as seen from the left side of the esophagus

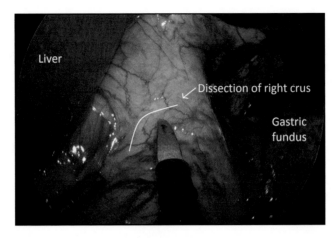

Fig. 7.3 Hiatal dissection viewed from the right. Note the access can be made via an incision in the peritoneum at the anterior border of the right crus above the hepatic branch of the vagus, rather than a pars flaccida (gastro-hepatic omentum) approach

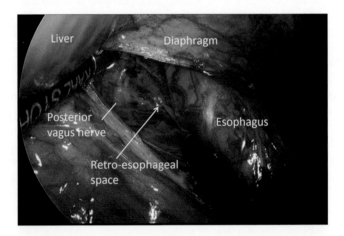

Fig. 7.4 Dissection is extended into the retro-esophageal space from the right side

mobilised by sharp and blunt dissection from the left, which makes dissection from the right side and subsequent encirclement considerably easier.

Division of the pars flaccida is not required to access the right crus. A small window can be made in tissue overlying the right crus above the hepatic branch of the vagus nerve, and dissection then proceeds down onto fascia and into the right hiatal space to complete dissection on that side (Figs. 7.3 and 7.4). This approach eliminates the possibility of a "slipped" fundoplication.

It is vital that the vagus nerves are identified and protected in the process of esophageal mobilisation, since damage to either can produce the long-term significant disabilities of gastroparesis (anterior vagus) and diarrhoea (posterior vagus). To do this, the esophagus should be mobilised on each side and posteriorly, before

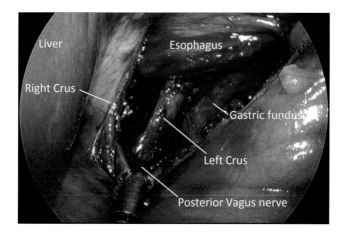

Fig. 7.5 The right and left hiatal crura are seen exposed behind the esophagus and retain their peritoneal covering. The posterior vagus nerve is not included in the wrap

being encircled with a retraction loop, and the anterior aspect gently mobilised last. *Anteriorly, the safest plane is in the loose areolar tissue anterior to the esophagus, since the anterior vagus nerve will remain in close proximity to the esophagus and thus is safe from dissection in this plane.*

With the esophagus slung, dissection can be performed using the harmonic scalpel posterior to the esophagus to create a space for the fundal wrap. Care must be employed to avoid injury to the posterior vagus nerve and to the stomach itself (Fig. 7.5).

Once this has been done, the esophagus can be mobilised more proximally by a combination of blunt and sharp dissection in order to increase intra-abdominal length. Esophageal dissection should be precise, carried out in tissue planes, and bloodless.

Closure of the Hiatus

Hiatal closure will be required in the majority cases. Recurrent herniation occurs firstly at the left posterior aspect of the hiatus, and a posterior herniation of the wrap is the first stage of failure [5]. It therefore makes sense that posterior closure of the hiatal pillars is important for structural integrity, with additional closure anteriorly in the larger defects. Sutures should be placed so as to incorporate the fascia overlying the hiatal pillars, as well as muscle, to ensure the most secure closure (Fig. 7.6). Since hiatal closure can cause post-operative dysphagia independent of the wrap, the closure should not be at all tight. There should be room for 2 blunt-nosed graspers to fit comfortably in the anterior aspect of the hiatus after completion of the hiatal repair and wrap.

In certain patients, such as those who are young and fit, without a hiatal hernia and with good muscular peri-hiatal tissue, a hiatal repair may not be necessary.

Since the left postero-lateral aspect of the hiatus is most vulnerable to late fundal herniation, the left phreno-esophageal ligament can be re-sutured to the esophagus

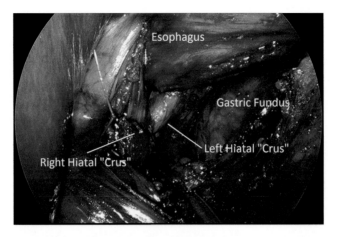

Fig. 7.6 Closure of the hiatal crura, as seen from the right side

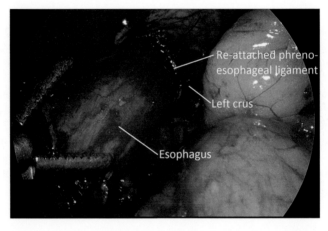

Fig. 7.7 Re-attachment of the crus to the esophagus, creating a 5-cm segment of abdominal esophagus

at this point to re-establish stability in this area, also giving approximately 5 cm of abdominal esophagus, prior to bougie insertion and formation of the wrap (Fig. 7.7). This can be done with a continuous suture from approximately 6 to 1 o'clock (3/0).

The Wrap

A modern Toupet fundoplication is a posterior partial wrap that can be from 180° (as was the original Toupet technique) up to 270°, with most centres opting for the 270° wrap. In Toupet's original wrap, the short gastric vessels were not divided, and so the posterior aspect of the fundus was drawn behind the esophagus to create the wrap.

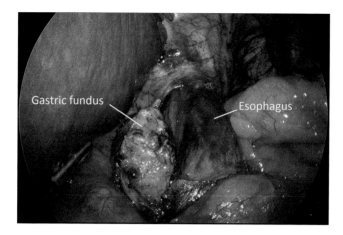

Fig. 7.8 The fundus is drawn behind the esophagus for the right side of the wrap. It sits in place comfortably without tension, or the need to be held prior to suturing

The wrap does not tend to "sit" well in position without being held in this circumstance. In setting up the wrap after division of short gastric vessels, it is important to "rotate" the fundus anti-clockwise as it is drawn behind the esophagus with the "pivot" being the angle of His. In this way, when the wrap is "set" before suturing, the divided short gastric vessels lie anteriorly along the fundus on the right side of the esophagus (Fig. 7.8). One must remember to loosen the omental retraction sutures beforehand. In this position, the wrap should sit comfortably and symmetrically without the need to be held prior to suturing.

Suturing the Wrap

Subsequent suturing should avoid incorporating the anterior vagus nerve, and the wrap should be attached to the hiatal margin as well as the esophagus. This suture is placed at approximately 10–11 o'clock to the right of the anterior vagus nerve and includes the esophagus, hiatus, and superior border of the wrap. A 46–52FG bougie is helpful in gauging tension and space and is still routinely used in our Unit. Generally, we use a continuous suture for the wrap attaching fundus to esophagus, the proximal attachment including the diaphragm. Interrupted sutures are also suitable. The first suture line attaches the right side of the wrap to the esophagus, and esophagus and diaphragm at the hiatus. The next suture to be placed attaches the wrap on the left side to the esophagus and crus at the "5 o'clock" position (Fig. 7.9). This suture functions as a "gastropexy" of stomach to the left crus. The next suture line finalises the wrap by attaching the left side of the wrap to the esophagus, the proximal suture incorporating the hiatus in similar fashion to the right side just described. One continues to fashion the left side of the wrap by attaching the fundus to the esophagus along a line approximately at the 1–2 o'clock position (Fig. 7.10).

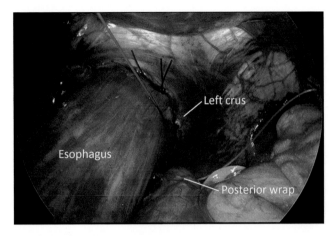

Fig. 7.9 Suture placement left posterior aspect to include crus, fundal wrap, and esophagus. This ensures fixation at the point where recurrent herniation is most likely to occur

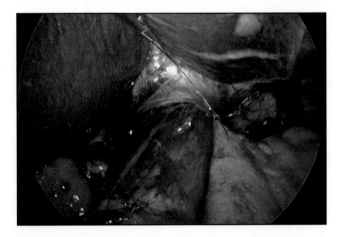

Fig. 7.10 The anchor suture is placed between 1 and 2 o'clock to commence the left side of the fundoplication

Finally, a single gastropexy suture is placed from the right side of the wrap to esophagus and right crus at the "7 o'clock" position. We regard stability of the wrap attached to the diaphragm as important in preventing later herniation and hiatal failure, hence the sutures placed at 5 and 7 o'clock to the crura described above, and thus form a gastropexy. The right posterior crural stitch is more easily done after the bougie is removed.

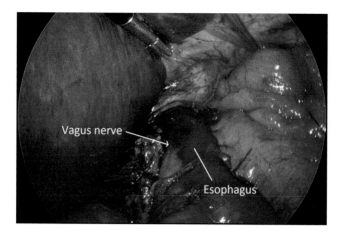

Fig. 7.11 The completed Toupet fundoplication

Final Inspection

It goes without saying that the final finished wrap should look symmetrical and sit comfortably without tension (Fig. 7.11). Such a fundoplication will usually work well. *A distorted or asymmetric wrap, or one that causes rotation to the esophagus, usually does not function appropriately and will need re-fashioning.* Blood loss should be negligible, and there should be minimal tissue trauma as sharp dissection in anatomic planes is possible in all aspects of the operation. The vagus nerves should remain intact and be subject to minimal handling or trauma.

After removal of the bougie, there should be space anteriorly to easily take the tips of two blunt-nosed laparoscopic graspers. *Note that post-operative dysphagia can be caused by a tight hiatus, particularly distressing in those who need to immediately resume oral medications (e.g., lung transplant patients), or those of borderline weight.* We would emphasize that the above approach to the Toupet operation is based on our own experience and works well for us. However, other approaches to the Toupet fundoplication are equally valid if they produce good clinical results.

Post-operative Care

Patients are commenced on a fluid diet after 6 h. The following day a soft food diet is commenced, which is maintained for 4 weeks post-operatively, and the intravenous line removed. This diet essentially excludes "chunky" foods such as solid meats and fruits (e.g., apple) and undercooked or raw vegetables. It also excludes doughy foods such as thick fresh bread, buns, and the like. If there is difficulty swallowing large-sized medications, these can be more easily taken on a spoon with custard or yoghurt. Troublesome post-operative dysphagia is rare following the Toupet operation. The soft food diet is almost universally well-tolerated. In our experience early reoperation or dilatation for dysphagia has been eliminated with use of the Toupet wrap.

Anaesthetic Aspects

All the usual preoperative assessments and planning apply in laparoscopic fundoplication. Monitoring is selected based on patient comorbidities. Invasive arterial pressure monitoring is added if the patient has significant cardiac comorbidity, or in cases of a large hiatus hernia, there may be cardiac compression effects that may need monitoring.

Specific Considerations for Fundoplication

The presence of GERD is managed by modified rapid sequence induction, or full rapid sequence induction if the patient has a major volume regurgitation problem. A cuffed endotracheal tube should always be used in fundoplication surgery.

The patient is positioned head-up, usually 10–15°, but if the lithotomy position is used this can offset the cardiovascular impact to a degree. With capnoperitoneum, one can vary the pressure, usually commencing with 12 mmHg but sometimes more. The usual caveats regarding cardiovascular effects and organ perfusion will apply. Sometimes capnoperitoneum induction can precipitate profound bradycardia with loss of blood pressure and cardiac output. This is quickly rectified by evacuation of the capnoperitoneum and administration of intravenous atropine. The operation may then proceed without danger.

Subcutaneous emphysema is sometimes observed, as gas tracks up through the mediastinum, and can appear dramatic but does not tend to cause obstruction of the airway. It usually only causes hypercarbia and resolves rapidly in the post-operative phase. It can be treated with masterful inactivity.

Occasionally, capnothorax can occur, which can come under tension. It is diagnosed by clinical examination, together with a change in the CO_2 waveform and ventilatory pressure change. Ultrasound examination is a useful tool to confirm the diagnosis (both the standard view and M mode are used). If there is compromise of the cardiovascular or respiratory systems, then communication with the surgeon regarding reducing or releasing abdominal CO_2 pressure is helpful. The capnothorax resolves rapidly after capnoperitoneum is released and does not usually require drainage. However, if it is diagnosed, one can expect worse than usual shoulder tip pain in the post-operative recovery ward.

The duration of fundoplication is operator-dependent and is usually around 1–1.5 h with a skilled surgeon. Patient warming remains important, using warmed fluid and a forced air warming device.

Usually a 46–54 Fr bougie is placed in the upper esophagus and advanced upon request from the surgeon as a guide for wrap tightness. *It is wise to "feel" the bougie through the upper and lower sphincters during advancement and observe it entering stomach on screen. While rare, perforation is a risk, but minimised with slow and careful advancement.*

Post-Operation

Post-operative Nausea and Vomiting Avoidance and Management

Nausea management begins preoperatively, including a full discussion with the patient. There are many successful approaches available. If there is a history of motion sickness, one can add a vestibular sedative e.g., cyclizine 50 mg, or low dose hyoscine hydrobromide 40 mg iv or 100 mg sc to granisetron 3 mg and dexamethasone 8 mg as prophylaxis. It is best to avoid N_2O.

In the Recovery Ward, it is helpful to prescribe three anti-emetics and instruct Recovery Nurses of a plan: usually prochlorperazine 12.5 mg Q4H prn, ondansetron 4 mg q4h prn, and droperidol 1–2 mg q4h prn to be used in that order. If breakthrough nausea occurs, a careful midazolam infusion can be useful (5 mg per hour by constant infusion) and will need enhanced observations or High Dependency Unit admission, or addition of haloperidol 5 mg iv. Avoidance of hypothermia, hypo or hyperglycaemia, and pain is helpful. *It is vital to avoid retching or vomiting, both from a patient comfort point of view and as it may risk damaging the repair.*

Analgesia

Port site and visceral pain is managed with intraoperative NSAID (if not contraindicated) and opioid. A pain protocol in the Recovery Ward is very helpful. If there is a history of Post-operative Nausea and Vomiting (PONV) with morphine, a fentanyl PCA is used as part of PONV management plan. Usually when on the surgical ward, patients need only prn (as required) subcutaneous opioid during the first day and then a switch to oral analgesia prior to discharge the next day.

Referred pain in the shoulder or neck is managed by education preoperatively and warm packs and acetaminophen iv. The use of warm insufflation gas and fully venting CO_2 at case end may reduce this referred pain. We tend not to give acetaminophen intraoperatively, saving it for use in the recovery ward.

Esophageal "spasm-like" pain (dull central chest pain, constant in nature, clearly distinct from abdominal pain or referred shoulder pain) occurs occasionally, more often in younger patients. If it occurs, there may be a need to exclude a cardiac cause by history and examination, ECG and if needed, serial serum troponin levels. Treatment is by reassurance, change in posture (often sitting upright and deep slow breathing exercise is helpful), and if the patient is sufficiently alert, sipping warm water.

Pharmacologic treatment options include hyoscine butylbromide, GTN, calcium channel blockers e.g., verapamil or glucagon. The effect of glucagon is quite short. These interventions may help, but often simple measures mentioned above are more useful. Gentle anxiolysis can also be useful e.g., Midazolam 1 mg iv as a bolus. It is wise to avoid excessive opioids as this does not settle esophageal pain well and are likely to cause over-sedation with exacerbation of post-operative nausea and vomiting and/or respiratory depression.

In summary, it is very useful to prepare the patient with a good understanding of what to expect. Manage problems as they arise intra-operatively and anticipate post-operative issues. The single most important point is patient preparation preoperatively.

Results

There is a large published literature documenting the short- and long-term results of the Toupet fundoplication [6–14]. In comparative studies, the Nissen fundoplication is usually the benchmark, based on its long established history in the surgical treatment of GERD, and it remains arguably the most popular fundoplication technique in use today. However, the operation can result in adverse side effects such as dysphagia and gas retention symptoms such as excessive bloating and flatus. This is why a number of clinical trials involving a reduced circumference wrap have been undertaken and published. In such trials, level one randomised controlled trials have the most validity since the influence of bias is reduced. Table 7.1 summarises a group of such trials involving comparison between theToupet and Nissen fundoplication techniques [6–14]. These trials can be analysed according to the factors that are most important to patients: safety, efficacy, longevity, and a low rate of side effects. It is most unusual these days for a patient to die as a result of antireflux surgery, so most studies have zero operative mortality.

As a general rule, the less the extent of the wrap, the fewer the side effects such as dysphagia and gas-bloat, but there is evidence that these lesser wraps risk higher

Table 7.1 Summary of results of randomised controlled trials comparing the Toupet and the Nissen fundoplications

Author	Year	Years F/U	No. of Patients	Reflux control	Dysphagia	Bloat/ flatus
Hagedorn**o	2002	11.5	110	Equal	↑ Nissen*	↑ Nissen
Mardani**o	2011	18	80	Equal	Equal	Equal
Chrysos	2003	1	33	Equal	↑ Nissen*	↑ Nissen
Guérin	2007	1 and 3	121	Equal	Equal	Equal
Booth	2008	1	127	Equal	↑ Nissen	Equal
Strate	2008	2	200	Equal	↑ Nissen	↑ Nissen
Shaw	2010	3–5	100	Equal	Equal	nr
Mickevicius	2013	5	129	Equal	Equal	Equal
Koch	2013	1	125	Equal	↑ Nissen	↑ Nissen

↑* early, equal > 1 year, ** Same trial, oOpen operations, nr = data not reported recurrence rates of reflux symptoms. However, the Toupet fundoplication seems to confer a similar degree of reflux control when compared to the Nissen fundoplication, which is durable for at least 18 years [7]. Along with this, there appears to be a reduced risk of post-operative dysphagia and gassy side effects, at least for the short and medium term.

A systematic review and meta-analysis of laparoscopic Nissen and Toupet fundoplications found a higher incidence of dysphagia and surgical reinterventions after the Nissen operation, but no differences in acid exposure, esophagitis, symptomatic recurrence, patient satisfaction, operating time, or complications [15]. The study found inability to belch and gas bloat to be more prevalent after the Nissen fundoplication. However, over the long term, perhaps after 5 years or more, the side effect profile of the Nissen and Toupet fundoplications appear to be comparable [7].

Randomised trials also demonstrate that in the presence of non-specific motility disorders, such as diminished amplitude and failed contractions, "tailoring" to a lesser degree of wrap is not needed in order to reduce the risk of post-operative dysphagia [10, 11, 16].

Our own results have been recorded prospectively since 1991 on a computerised database where only completed patient data are considered in analyses and correspond to the introduction of the laparoscopic approach. Until the year 2000, the Nissen fundoplication was the operation of choice in our hands, with the Toupet employed for patients with deficient esophageal motility (motility and pH studies were mandatory then, selective now). As a result of the influential publication by Hagedorn et al. [6] comparing the Nissen and Toupet with 10-year follow-up results showing reduced dysphagia and gassy side effects with the Toupet procedure, our practice changed to employing the Toupet operation as our preferred primary operation for GERD. Between 1991 and 2008 (16 years), 5080 laparoscopic fundoplications were undertaken in our surgical unit, 3982 as primary operations for GERD, 627 accompanying para-esophageal hiatal hernia repair, and 471 re-do operations. Of the primary operations for reflux, 2549 were Nissen fundoplications and 1128 were Toupet operations undertaken by 3 surgeons. There was no mortality and a current re-operation rate of 3 % at 15 years follow-up.

All patients were assessed preoperatively using the DeMeester score for reflux symptoms [17], then repeated at 1, 3, 5, and 10 years (Tables 7.2, 7.3, 7.4, 7.5). This was accompanied by a gastrointestinal symptom questionnaire, addressing a range

Table 7.2 The DeMeester score for symptoms of GERD [17]

Score	Definition (abbreviated from original)
0	No symptoms
1	Occasional, brief episodes
2	Frequent symptoms >2/week. Postural. Daily anti-secretory agents (episodes of bolus obstruction requiring liquids to clear in cases of dysphagia)
3	Nocturnal symptoms, PPI dependence, poor quality of life (episodes of bolus obstruction requiring hospitalisation in cases of dysphagia)

Table 7.3 Comparison between the Nissen and Toupet fundoplications in controlling heartburn over a 10-year follow-up period using the DeMeester score

Heartburn										
DeMeester score	Nissen %					Toupet %				
N	Pre 2549	1Y 2220	3Y 1873	5Y 1516	10Y 596	Pre 1128	1Y 876	3Y 556	5Y 321	10Y 55
0/1 %	12	94	93	90	89	18	93	92	89	87
2 %	16	4	5	6	7	24	5	6	9	11
3 %	72	2	2	4	4	58	2	2	1	2

Ratings 0 and 1 are combined for ease of display

Table 7.4 Comparison between the Nissen and Toupet fundoplications in controlling regurgitation over a 10-year follow-up period using the DeMeester score

Regurgitation										
DeMeester score	Nissen %					Toupet %				
N	Pre 2549	1Y 2220	3Y 1873	5Y 1516	10Y 596	Pre 1128	1Y 876	3Y 556	5Y 321	10Y 55
0/1 %	23	94	93	90	89	16	93	92	90	86
2 %	31	4	5	6	7	31	5	6	9	12
3 %	46	2	2	4	4	53	2	2	1	2

Table 7.5 Comparison between the Nissen and Toupet fundoplications in controlling dysphagia over a 10-year follow-up period using the DeMeester score

Dyaphagia										
DeMeester score	Nissen %					Toupet %				
N	Pre 2549	1Y 2220	3Y 1873	5Y 1516	10Y 596	Pre 1128	1Y 876	3Y 556	5Y 321	10Y 55
0/1 %	81	90	91	91	90	80	92	92	93	87
2 %	16	8	7	7	9	17	7	7	6	9
3 %	3	2	2	2	1	53	1	1	2	4

of gastrointestinal side effects. Reflux control (heartburn, regurgitation) was similar between the Nissen and Toupet fundoplications out to 10 years post-operatively. There was no difference in dysphagia rates between the operations at each time point, using the DeMeester scale, and overall preoperative dysphagia was actually reduced by both of the operations ($p < 0.001$).

For gastrointestinal side effects, there was reduced ability to belch at 1 and 5 years after the Nissen operation ($p < 0.001$), and reduced nausea and flatus at 1 year for the Toupet ($p < 0.001$) (Fisher's "exact" test), but no difference at 3, 5, and 10 years. Our results are in concert generally with the published literature: the Toupet fundoplication is as effective in controlling reflux over time as the Nissen operation, but generally with less risk of gassy side effects and dysphagia in the first few years after operation.

Conclusions

Our view, based on the published literature and our experience, is that the choice of operation for GERD is not as important as careful selection of patients, realistic and in-depth discussion with the patient preoperatively, meticulous surgical and anaesthetic technique, together with ongoing post-operative care until early side effects have resolved. Communication is time-consuming, but is important to the success of the procedure.

We have also established a long-term collaborative and trusted working relationship with our Gastroenterologists and referring Internists and regard this as essential in order to provide a balanced treatment pathway for patients as their GERD evolves over time.

We do not have a perfect operation for GERD. There will always be a failure rate over time, and side effects will still occur. However, surgical management is far more successful than medical therapy and endoscopic techniques for controlling severe GERD disease over the long-term [18].

Acknowledgements Dr Douglas McEwan, MB. BS. FANZCA. For his input on anaesthesia tips for laparoscopic fundoplication. Colleagues Dr Mark Smithers, Dr Andrew Barbour, Dr Iain Thompson.

References

1. Toupet A. Technique d'esophago-gastroplastie avec phreno-gastropexie dans la cure radicales des hernies hiatales et comme complement de l'operation de Heller dans les cardiospasmes. Mem Acad Chir. 1963;89:394–9.
2. Katkhouda N, Khalil MR, Manhas S, Grant S, Velmahos GC, Umbach TW, Kaiser AM. André Toupet: surgeon technician par excellence. Ann Surg. 2002;235(4):591–9.
3. Engström C, Jamieson GG, Devitt PG, Watson DI. Meta-analysis of two randomized controlled trials to identify long-term symptoms after division of the short gastric vessels during Nissen fundoplication. Br J Surg. 2011;98(8):1063–7.
4. DeMeester SR. Laparoscopic para-esophageal hernia repair: critical steps and adjunct techniques to minimize recurrence. Surg Laparosc Endosc Percutan Tech. 2013;23(5):429–35.
5. Byrne JP, Smithers BM, Nathanson LK, Martin I, Ong HS, Gotley DC. Symptomatic and functional outcome after laparoscopic reoperation for failed antireflux surgery. Br J Surg. 2005;92(8):996–1001.
6. Hagedorn C, Lönroth H, Rydberg L, Ruth M, Lundell L. Long-term efficacy of total (Nissen-Rossetti) and posterior partial (Toupet) fundoplication: results of a randomized clinical trial. J Gastrointest Surg. 2002;6(4):540–5.
7. Mardani J, Lundell L, Engström C. Total or posterior partial fundoplication in the treatment of GERD: results of a randomized trial after 2 decades of follow-up. Ann Surg. 2011;253(5):875–8.
8. Chrysos E, Tsiaoussis J, Zoras OJ, Athanasakis E, Mantides A, Katsamouris A, Xynos E. Laparoscopic surgery for gastroesophageal reflux disease patients with impaired esophageal peristalsis: total or partial fundoplication? J Am Coll Surg. 2003;197(1):8–15.
9. Guérin E, Bétroune K, Closset J, Mehdi A, Lefèbvre JC, Houben JJ, Gelin M, Vaneukem P, El Nakadi I. Nissen versus Toupet fundoplication: results of a randomized and multicenter trial. Surg Endosc. 2007;21(11):1985–90.

10. Booth MI, Stratford J, Jones L, Dehn TC. Randomized clinical trial of laparoscopic total (Nissen) versus posterior partial (Toupet) fundoplication for gastro-oesophageal reflux disease based on preoperative oesophageal manometry. Br J Surg. 2008;95(1):57–63.

11. Strate U, Emmermann A, Fibbe C, Layer P, Zornig C. Laparoscopic fundoplication: Nissen versus Toupet two-year outcome of a prospective randomized study of 200 patients regarding preoperative esophageal motility. Surg Endosc. 2008;22(1):21–30.

12. Shaw JM, Bornman PC, Callanan MD, Beckingham IJ, Metz DC. Long-term outcome of laparoscopic Nissen and laparoscopic Toupet fundoplication for gastroesophageal reflux disease: a prospective, randomized trial. Surg Endosc. 2010;24(4):924–32.

13. Mickevičius A, Endzinas Ž, Kiudelis M, Jonaitis L, Kupčinskas L, Pundzius J, Maleckas A. Influence of wrap length on the effectiveness of Nissen and Toupet fundoplications: 5-year results of prospective, randomized study. Surg Endosc. 2013;27(3):986–91. doi:10.1007/s00464-012-2550-7.

14. Koch OO, Kaindlstorfer A, Antoniou SA, Luketina RR, Emmanuel K, Pointner R. Comparison of results from a randomized trial 1 year after laparoscopic Nissen and Toupet fundoplications. Surg Endosc. 2013;27(7):2383–90.

15. Broeders JA, Roks DJ, Ahmed Ali U, Draaisma WA, Smout AJ, Hazebroek EJ. Laparoscopic anterior versus posterior fundoplication for gastroesophageal reflux disease: systematic review and meta-analysis of randomized clinical trials. Ann Surg. 2011;254(1):39–47. Review.

16. Rydberg L, Ruth M, Abrahamsson H, Lundell L. Tailoring of anti-reflux surgery: A randomised clinical trial. World J Surg. 1999;23(6):612–8.

17. Johnson LF, Demeester TR. Twenty-four-hour pH monitoring of the distal esophagus. A quantitative measure of gastroesophageal reflux. Am J Gastroenterol. 1974;62(4):325–32.

18. Lundell L, Miettinen P, Myrvold HE, Hatlebakk JG, Wallin L, Malm A, Sutherland I, Walan A, Nordic GORD Study Group. Seven-year follow-up of a randomized clinical trial comparing proton-pump inhibition with surgical therapy for reflux oesophagitis. Br J Surg. 2007;94(2):198–203.

Chapter 8
Anterior Partial Fundoplication

David I. Watson and Björn Törnqvist

Rationale for Anterior Partial Fundoplication

Although Nissen fundoplication undoubtedly offers effective treatment for gastro-esophageal reflux disease [1, 2], postoperative dysphagia and gas-related symptoms have encouraged modifications which aim to reduce the risk of side effects, including the development of partial wraps [2–4]. When constructing either a posterior partial fundoplication or a Nissen fundoplication, the gastric fundus is placed behind the distal esophagus, and this can lift the distal esophagus anteriorly and angulate it at the gastro-esophageal junction. It has been hypothesized that these factors might contribute to dysphagia and other unwanted side effects. Construction of an anterior partial fundoplication places the gastric fundus in front of the intra-abdominal esophagus and does not push the gastro-esophageal junction forward or angulate the distal esophagus to the extent that occurs with the other fundoplication types. This results in a more anatomically correct position, with theoretically less negative side effects.

In patients with achalasia, a Dor fundoplication, an anterior partial fundoplication variant, is often added to surgical cardiomyotomy to minimize postoperative reflux issues [5]. The division of the lower esophageal sphincter, together with the lack of esophageal peristalsis in achalasia, results in a highly refluxogenic situation, and it

D.I. Watson, MBBS, MD, FRACS, FAHMS (✉)
Flinders University Department of Surgery, Flinders Medical Centre,
Adelaide, South Australia, Australia
e-mail: david.watson@flinders.edu.au

B. Törnqvist, M.D., Ph.D.
Department of Upper Gastrointestinal Surgery, Karolinska University Hospital,
Stockholm 14186, Sweden

© Springer International Publishing Switzerland 2016
R.W. Aye, J.G. Hunter (eds.), *Fundoplication Surgery*,
DOI 10.1007/978-3-319-25094-6_8

is widely accepted that an anterior partial fundoplication is a good treatment option for these patients, providing appropriate reflux control and a low risk of side effects. As anterior partial fundoplication is effective in this difficult patient group, it is logical to use it more broadly as an alternative to Nissen fundoplication in patients undergoing surgeryfor gastro-esophageal reflux in whom it is desirable to minimize the risk of post-fundoplication side effects. Examples include high risk situations such as patients with reflux and an aperistaltic esophagus [6], patients with atypical reflux symptoms, e.g., throat symptoms [7], and "challenging" patients [8]. If operating on the latter groups, an anterior partial fundoplication offers reflux control and an operation that minimizes the risk of adding new post-fundoplication problems.

While we first applied an anterior partial fundoplication in a subgroup of patients for whom we aimed to control reflux but also minimize adverse side effects, ongoing experience, randomized trials, and late follow-up of large prospective case series have all encouraged broader application of this approach to the majority of patients with gastro-esophageal reflux patient [9–11], in whom for long time the Nissen fundoplication has been considered to be the gold-standard procedure.

Several variants of anterior partial fundoplication have been described—90°, 120°, and 180° anterior partial fundoplications, with the extent of anchorage of the fundoplication to the right side of the hiatal rim varying across these approaches [12–14]. Six randomized controlled trials have compared Nissen vs. anterior 180° partial fundoplication [11, 15–19]. The first trial was conducted in our institution. One hundred and seven patients with gastro-esophageal reflux disease were randomly assigned to Nissen vs. anterior 180° partial fundoplication and results have been reported at 6-months, 5-years, and 10 years of follow-up. At 6-months, equivalent control of reflux was seen, but patients who had undergone anterior fundoplication had significantly less dysphagia for solid food and were more likely to be satisfied with the clinical outcome [15]. *Analyses at 5 years confirmed the early outcome of less side effects after anterior 180° partial fundoplication, although this was offset by slightly better reflux control following Nissen fundoplication [16]. After 10 years, however, there were no significant differences for reflux symptoms, side effects, and overall satisfaction [11]. Similar outcomes have been identified in the other randomized trials. Overall reoperation rates were lower following anterior 180° partial fundoplication, compared to the Nissen procedure, principally due to a lower risk of dysphagia and hiatus hernia following anterior partial fundoplication.*

In a trial enrolling 161 patients, Baigrie et al. [17] also reported similar reflux control and less dysphagia 2 years after anterior 180° partial fundoplication. Cao et al. [18] enrolled 100 patients and also found equivalent reflux control at 5 years, but with less flatulence after anterior 180° partial fundoplication. A recent meta-analysis [20] concluded similar control of reflux symptoms, PPI use, and patient satisfaction, but less dysphagia and gas-related symptoms after anterior 180° partial fundoplication compared to Nissen at 1 and 5 years.

For anterior 90° and anterior 120° partial fundoplication, the supporting data is less robust [21]. Two randomized trials have compared anterior 90° partial vs. Nissen fundoplication [22–24]. At early follow-up (6 months), less side effects were seen following the anterior 90° partial fundoplication, but traded off against a slightly higher incidence of recurrent reflux [22]. At later follow-up to 5 years, side effects and overall satisfaction were similar for both fundoplication types, but reflux was more common following anterior 90° partial fundoplication [23].

Based on this data, our preference when constructing a partial fundoplication to treat gastro-esophageal reflux is to construct an anterior 180° partial fundoplication, and not one of the lesser variants. *From a practical perspective, in clinical practice, patients presentingforsurgery for gastro-esophageal reflux in whom work-up with esophageal manometry demonstrates normal or relatively normal esophageal motility are involved in a discussion about the risks of side effects vs. the risk of recurrent reflux after anterior 180° vs. Nissen fundoplication, and then encouraged to choose the type of fundoplication which best fits their expectations. For patients with poor esophageal motility, and patients who are thought to be at significant risk of not tolerating side effects, an anterior 180° partial fundoplication would always be recommended.* Currently, in the authors' practice approximately 80–90 % of individuals undergoing surgery for gastro-esophageal reflux undergo an anterior 180° partial fundoplication, with the remainder opting for a Nissen fundoplication [10].

Surgical Technique for Anterior 180° Partial Fundoplication

When constructing an anterior partial fundoplication, the key steps are to reduce and repair any hiatal hernia, stabilize and maintain a length of esophagus within the abdomen, and create a flap valve by anchoring the anterior fundus across the front of the esophagus. To achieve a good long-term outcome, this anatomy needs to remain stable for the remainder of the patient's life. *When constructing an anterior 180° partial fundoplication, the gastric fundus is sutured to the diaphragmatic hiatus, and this step contributes to the long-term stability of the fundoplication.* The lesser degrees of anterior partial fundoplication, 90° and 120°, suture the fundus to the anterior wall of the esophagus, rather than to the right hiatal pillar, and this might allow unravelling of the wrap with time, contributing to an apparently higher rate of recurrent reflux.

In addition, to ensure long-term stability of the fundoplication and the intra-abdominal position of the gastro-esophageal junction, sufficiently large bites of tissue must be taken when each suture is placed through the wall of the stomach, the esophagus, and the hiatal rim. Initially, there is a tendency for surgeons to be cautious and to only take superficial bites of the critical structures, especially the esophageal wall. *The fear of placing the suture needle too deep within the wall of the esophagus should be resisted, as firm anchorage of the esophagus within the abdomen is critical to long-term success.*

Positioning and Port Placement

The patient is positioned head-up with the legs extended in stirrups or split in extension, so that the operating surgeon can stand between the patient's legs, with an assistant on the patient's left side. An 11-mm port is placed supraumbilically for a

Fig. 8.1 Port placement.
(*A*) 11-mm port for
laparoscope. (*B*) 5-mm
port for surgeon's left
hand. (*C*) Nathanson liver
retractor. (*D*) 11-mm port
for surgeon's right hand,
passage of suture needles,
and placement of tape to
retract esophagus. (*E*)
5-mm port for assistant's
retracting instrument

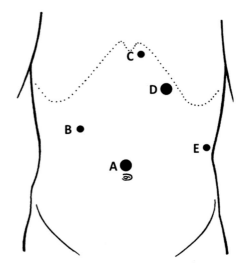

30° laparoscope. The author's preference is to use a supraumbilical open entry technique, although this can be modified to a left upper quadrant optical entry approach if midline adhesions are anticipated. Under vision, other ports are placed; one 5-mm port is placed in the right midclavicular line approximately 5 cm below the costal margin. An 11-mm port is placed immediately subcostal in the left midclavicular line and used as the main surgical working port. A 5-mm port is placed subcostally in the left anterior axillary line for use by the assistant, and a Nathanson liver retractor is placed via a 5-mm sub-xiphoid incision to expose the upper stomach and the gastro-esophageal junction (Fig. 8.1).

Hiatal Dissection and Repair

Dissection commences by exposing the outer aspect of the right hiatal pillar by bluntly opening the lesser omentum above and below the hepatic branch of the vagus. This is readily achieved using two laparoscopic grasping/dissecting instruments to pick up and separate the avascular semitransparent area of the lesser omentum first below the hepatic branch and then above. The nerve is deliberately spared in most cases, but can be divided if it precludes safe esophageal dissection or suture placement.

In the absence of a large hiatus hernia, the hiatus is first dissected anteriorly on the right side. Dissection should remain approximately 5 mm inside the hiatal rim to ensure the fascial coverings of the crural muscle are preserved. Our preference is to use two grasping/dissecting instruments to bluntly dissect the hiatus, with the diathermy hook used only occasionally in selected cases. If dissecting in the correct plane, the muscle at the hiatal rim will remain covered by its fascia, and the dissection will be virtually bloodless. Other energy sources such as ultrasonic shears are unnecessary, extend the length of the operation, add cost, and increase the risk of injury to the esophageal wall.

Dissection is next extended across the front of the hiatus to the left pillar and downwards posteriorly along the left pillar edge. The peritoneal reflection overlying the left pillar does not overlie the phreno-esophageal ligament, but sits more laterally and is easily pushed or stripped off the under-surface of the diaphragm to partly mobilize the gastric fundus and expose the edge of the left pillar and phreno-esophageal ligament for dissection in a similar fashion to the right side. If a large hiatus hernia is present, then the hernia sac should be fully dissected and removed from the thorax before any further dissection of the esophagus is undertaken. An energy source is usually needed for dissection of the sac from the hiatal edge, but for this maneuver a diathermy hook suffices and allows accurate dissection.

The distal esophagus is dissected after fully dissecting the hiatal rim. It is mobilized by gentle blunt dissection using the ends of the two closed grasping instruments in a closed fashion. A plane is then developed behind the esophagus from right to left. Blind dissection or the use of an energy source behind the esophagus is avoided to minimize the risk of esophageal perforation. An atraumatic grasper is passed behind the distal esophagus from right to left, and a long linen tape is then passed via the 11 mm left upper port to the atraumatic grasper, pulled behind the esophagus, and then passed back to the surgeon's right hand instrument and pulled out through the left upper port (Fig. 8.2). This port is then removed and re-sited so that the tape runs across the abdominal wall outside the shaft of the 11-mm port. Traction can then be placed on the tape externally and tension maintained externally using an artery clip across the tape. Dissection then continues behind the esophagus until both hiatal pillars are well-displayed and the left pillar is clearly visible from

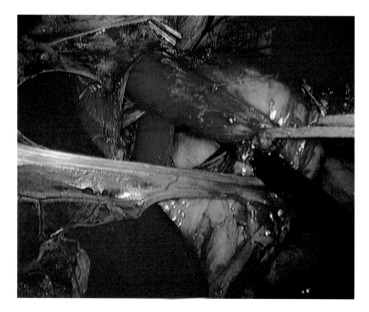

Fig. 8.2 Dissected esophageal hiatus. The hepatic branch of the vagus nerve remains intact. A linen tape is retracting the gastro-esophageal junction

behind the esophagus, and an adequate space is available for suturing. During these steps, the posterior vagus nerve is seen and dissected away from the posterior aspect of the esophagus, so that it can be placed posterior to the hiatal repair sutures.

The hiatus is repaired posteriorly by approximating the left and right pillars using 2-0 non-resorbable, monofilament sutures. One to three sutures are usually sufficient, and care should be taken not to narrow the hiatus too much, as overly narrowing this space might cause dysphagia (Figs. 8.3 and 8.4). The tape is removed after repairing the hiatus.

Construction of the Anterior 180° Partial Fundoplication

The anterior part of the fundus is slid laterally to the right across the front of the distal esophagus, without dividing the short gastric vessels, and then sutured in place. Key steps for this maneuver require the assistant to pull the pericardial fat pad downwards with a grasper, thereby reducing the gastro-esophageal junction 4–5 cm into the abdomen. A piece of the upper part of the anterior gastric fundus, not more than 1/4–1/3 of the distance from the gastro-esophageal junction to the greater curvature of the fundus, is manipulated and slid in front of the distal esophagus to form a tension-free fundoplication (Fig. 8.5). This is best achieved using two grasping instruments, and the fundus is slid laterally (not folded across) to the right to cover the distal esophagus. The position of the fundus should be checked carefully before

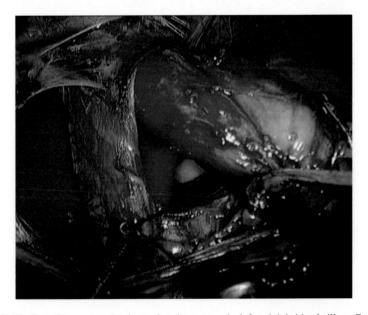

Fig. 8.3 The first of two sutures has been placed to appose the left and right hiatal pillars. Generous "bites" of the muscles and facial coverings are taken to ensure the repair is adequate

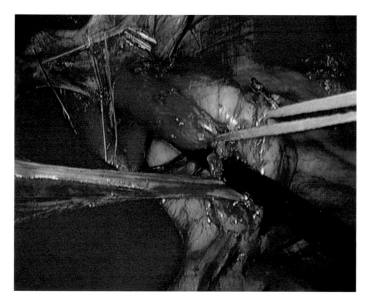

Fig. 8.4 Repaired hiatus. Two sutures have been placed and the hiatus has been narrowed. When suturing the hiatal pillars behind the esophagus, the repair should not be overly tight

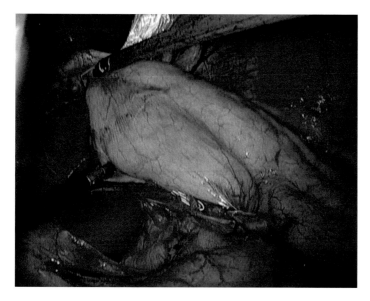

Fig. 8.5 The anterior fundus is slid laterally to the patient's right so that it sits loosely across the front of the esophagus and the esophageal hiatus. The first suture will be placed through the piece of stomach held by the lower grasping instrument

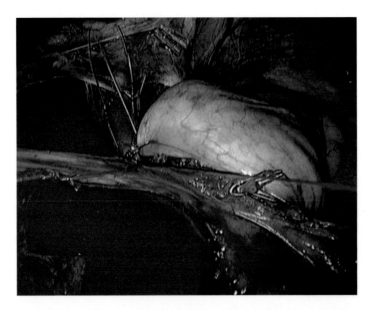

Fig. 8.6 The first suture anchors the fundus to the esophagus and the hiatal rim. Note the clips seen in an aberrant inferior left phrenic artery which has been divided to improve access

commencing suturing. It should sit loosely across the esophagus and the hiatus, and there should be no lines of tension extending out to the splenic hilum. It is important to stress that the stomach is slid over the front of the esophagus in a lateral direction, not folded across from left to right like turning a page in a book. If the stomach is folded across, the lateral fundus will only reach the right hiatal pillar under tension, and this will then demand division of the short gastric blood vessels to loosen that aspect of the fundus. When the correct piece of fundus is used, division of these vessels is unnecessary.

Generally, five sutures are used to secure the fundoplication. The first suture is critical as it sets up the rest of the fundoplication, and if correctly placed, all other sutures follow easily into the correct positions. This first suture anchors the fundus to the esophagus and the right hiatal pillar (Fig. 8.6). The next two sutures also include all three structures, and the final two sutures attach the fundus to the anterior hiatal rim to close the space anterior to the esophagus. The first suture includes the folded anterior fundus, the postero-lateral part of the distal esophagus (at least 2 cm above the gastro-esophageal junction), and the right hiatal pillar approximately at the same level as the previous most anterior hiatal repair suture. All sutures should include "generous" pieces of the relevant structures, and for the gastric fundus and the esophagus, they should be nearly full-thickness in depth. Including an equally "generous" piece of fascia-covered muscle maximizes the likelihood of a stable long-lasting fundoplication.

The second and third sutures are placed sequentially above the first suture, working anteriorly along the edge of the right hiatal pillar, and include the gastric

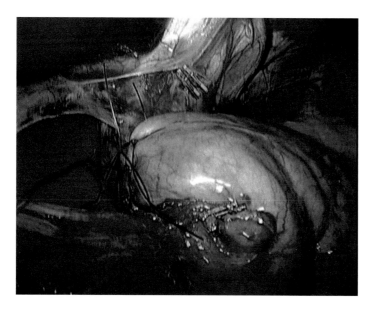

Fig. 8.7 Three sutures have been placed to secure the fundus and esophagus to the right hiatal pillar. These sutures fix the gastro-esophageal junction below the diaphragm and anchor the wrap

fundus, the right lateral esophagus, and the right hiatal rim (Fig. 8.7). These sutures are placed approximately 5–7 mm apart. Accurate placement of these sutures ensures a stable 3–4 cm length of intra-abdominal esophagus, and a fundoplication that is well-anchored to the hiatal rim, as well as a stable flap valve.

Finally, two "crown" stitches are placed to close the space between the esophagus and the hiatal rim anteriorly and on the anterolateral left side. These sutures do not include the wall of the esophagus, but close the hiatus by anchoring the edge of the folded fundus to the cranial portion of the hiatal rim at the 11 and 1–2 o'clock positions (Fig. 8.8).

Tips, Cautionary Tales, and Other Considerations

- *Suturing the left side of the esophagus to the adjacent gastric fundus is not necessary to accentuate the angle of His during anterior 180° partial fundoplication. Sliding the anterior fundus across the front of the esophagus and anchoring it to the right hiatal pillar creates a flap valve and accentuates the angle of His. Suturing the left side of the esophagus to adjacent gastric fundus limits the mobility of the gastric fundus and makes selection of the correct piece of the fundus for construction of the fundus more difficult.*
- *In overweight and obese patients, a satisfactory fundoplication can still be constructed, but excessive amounts of adipose tissue in the region of the esophageal*

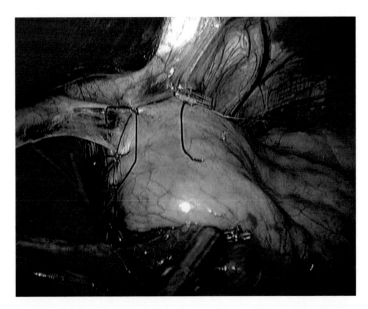

Fig. 8.8 Two additional "crown" sutures have been placed to close the anterior hiatus and complete the anterior 180° partial fundoplication

hiatus make dissection difficult, and a fatty liver reduces the operating space. Tilting the operating table up to 30° head up and the use of a Nathanson liver retractor facilitate adequate exposure. If only part of the operative field is initially visible, concentrate on the visible portion and adjust progressively the position of the liver retractor to maximize exposure of the area required for each step. The outcome for this type of fundoplication in obese patients is similar to the outcome for thinner patients [25].

- *The situation of a giant hiatus hernia with an intrathoracic stomach represents an increasingly larger component of the workload in most Western case-series. If encountered, the focus should initially be on dissecting the hernia sac from the chest rather than repositioning the stomach from the mediastinum. Dissecting 5–10 mm inside the edge of the hiatal defect reduces the risk of exposing bare muscle at the hiatal rim and ensures dissection does not make the defect larger and more difficult to close. An anterior 180° partial fundoplication can be added after hiatal repair. To prevent angulation of the esophagus and minimize dysphagia, the first fundoplication sutures should be placed through the right hiatal pillar at the same level as the most anterior hiatal repair suture, and the operation then continues as described above.*
- *Vascular injury can occur if the surgeon is unaware of the proximity of major vascular structures to the esophagus and the hiatal rim. Injury to the Inferior Vena Cava (IVC) is more likely when a large hiatus hernia is present, as the distance from the IVC to the edge of the right hiatal pillar can be less than 10 mm. Bluntly opening the avascular part of the lesser omentum below the hepatic vagal branch facilitates safe early identification of this vessel and*

dissection can be directed away from it at a safe distance. The use of energy sources such as ultrasonic shears to open the lesser omentum increases the risk of injury to the IVC and should be avoided at this stage.

- Theleft inferior phrenic arteryarises from the left gastric artery and runs aberrantly along the edge of right hiatal pillar in approximately 5–10 % of individuals. When located in this position, this vessel should be ligated or clipped, and then divided to adequately open the right anterolateral aspect of the esophageal hiatus. Care should be taken to look for this vessel before hiatal dissection commences. The vessel is easily seen, but will be injured if not ligated early.

- Theaorta lies posteriorto the hiatus, and the left hiatal pillar can be thin as it overlies this vessel. The aorta is at risk when placing the first suture through the left hiatal pillar for posterior hiatal repair. If arterial bleeding is encountered when placing this suture, the needle should be withdrawn and pressure applied for 5 min. Further intervention is rarely required.

- Theesophageal hiatuscan be dissected efficiently using 2 grasping instruments and a blunt dissection technique. The key is to dissect in the correct plane. The correct plane is bloodless. If bleeding is encountered, dissection is probably not in the correct plane and should be redirected. Energy sources are rarely needed unless a very large hiatus hernia is present. If required, the diathermy hook is sufficient for accurate dissection. Ultrasonic shears are general unhelpful, unless dividing short gastric blood vessels. All energy sources should be avoided behind theesophagusto minimize the risk of damage to the esophageal wall.

Postoperative Care

Patients commence oral fluids on the same day as surgery and pureed food the next day. Opiates should be avoided following surgery and a serotonin 5-HT$_3$ receptor antagonist (e.g., ondansetron) is routinely administered intraoperatively to minimize the risk of postoperative vomiting. A barium swallow X-ray is performed routinely at the first postoperative day to check the postoperative anatomy. Occasionally (<2 %), an acute para-esophageal hiatus hernia is seen, and this is easily repaired within a few days of the original surgery. The patient is usually discharged by the second postoperative day, and a pureed diet is continued for 4 weeks, after which the diet is graded back to normal over 4–8 weeks. Strenuous activity and lifting heavy objects should be avoided for 4 weeks to prevent disruption of the repair.

Outcomes

Late outcomes at 10 years follow-up following laparoscopic anterior 180° partial fundoplication have been determined in two follow-up studies from our department [9, 11]. Ninety-one to ninety-three percent of patients reported a good overall outcome at late follow-up, with good reflux control maintained long-term in the majority of patients—80 % report no heartburn, 13 % mild occasional symptoms, and 7 % report significant reflux symptoms at late follow-up. Proton pump inhibitor use was seen in 27 % of patients at 10 years follow-up, compared to 19 % following Nissen fundoplication, but only 1/3 of medication usage was for recurrent reflux. Troublesome dysphagia was rare at late follow-up and no patients required late revision surgery for this issue. Some bloating symptoms were reported in 29 % of individuals, but these symptoms were generally mild. Eighty-five percent of individuals retained the ability to belch effectively. The surgical revision rate across 10 years follow-up following anterior 180° partial fundoplication was 3.1 %, with revision for recurrent reflux undertaken in 2.4 % of individuals, and hiatus hernia in 0.5 %.

Conclusion

Anterior 180° partial fundoplication yields excellent long-term outcomes in patients undergoing surgery for gastro-esophageal reflux, with good reflux control, a reduced risk of side effects compared to the Nissen procedure, and excellent overall satisfaction with the surgical outcome. This procedure is simple to perform and requires minimal instrumentation. Additional steps such as division of the short gastric blood vessels and the use of expensive energy sources unnecessarily complicate the procedure. Understanding the perihiatal anatomy facilitates accurate dissection and correct suture placement to stabilize the gastro-esophageal junction and create a loose flap valve, which covers the anterior aspect of the intra-abdominal esophagus to ensure a good outcome.

References

1. Kelly JJ, Watson DI, Chin KF, et al. Laparoscopic Nissen fundoplication: clinical outcomes at 10 years. J Am Coll Surg. 2007;205:570–5.
2. Catarci M, Gentileschi P, Papi C, et al. Evidence-based appraisal of antireflux fundoplication. Ann Surg. 2004;239:325–37.
3. Varin O, Velstra B, De Sutter S, Ceelen W. Total vs partial fundoplication in the treatment of gastroesophageal reflux disease: a meta-analysis. Arch Surg. 2009;144:273–8.
4. Broeders JA, Mauritz FA, Ahmed Ali U, et al. Systematic review and meta-analysis of laparoscopic Nissen (posterior total) versus Toupet (posterior partial) fundoplication for gastro-oesophageal reflux disease. Br J Surg. 2010;97:1318–30.
5. Chen Z, Bessell JR, Chew A, Watson DI. Laparoscopic cardiomyotomy for achalasia: clinical outcomes beyond 5 years. J Gastrointest Surg. 2010;14:594–600.
6. Watson DI, Jamieson GG, Bessell JR, Devitt PG. Laparoscopic fundoplication in patients with an aperistaltic esophagus and gastroesophageal reflux. Dis Esophagus. 2006;19:94–8.
7. Ratnasingam D, Irvine T, Thompson SK, Watson DI. Laparoscopic antireflux surgery in patients with throat symptoms: a word of caution. World J Surg. 2011;35:342–8.
8. O'Boyle CJ, Watson DI, DeBeaux AC, Jamieson GG. Preoperative prediction of long-term outcome following laparoscopic fundoplication. ANZ J Surg. 2002;72:471–5.

9. Chen Z, Thompson SK, Jamieson GG, et al. Anterior 180-degree partial fundoplication: a 16-year experience with 548 patients. J Am Coll Surg. 2011;212:827–34.
10. Engstrom C, Cai W, Irvine T, et al. Twenty years of experience with laparoscopic antireflux surgery. Br J Surg. 2012;99:1415–21.
11. Cai W, Watson DI, Lally CJ, et al. Ten-year clinical outcome of a prospective randomized clinical trial of laparoscopic Nissen versus anterior 180(degrees) partial fundoplication. Br J Surg. 2008;95:1501–5.
12. Krysztopik RJ, Jamieson GG, Devitt PG, Watson DI. A further modification of fundoplication. 90 degrees anterior fundoplication. Surg Endosc. 2002;16:1446–51.
13. Gatenby PA, Bright T, Watson DI. Anterior 180 degrees partial fundoplication--how I do it. J Gastrointest Surg. 2012;16:2297–303.
14. Watson A, Jenkinson LR, Ball CS, et al. A more physiological alternative to total fundoplication for the surgical correction of resistant gastro-oesophageal reflux. Br J Surg. 1991;78:1088–94.
15. Watson DI, Jamieson GG, Pike GK, et al. Prospective randomized double-blind trial between laparoscopic Nissen fundoplication and anterior partial fundoplication. Br J Surg. 1999;86:123–30.
16. Ludemann R, Watson DI, Jamieson GG, et al. Five-year follow-up of a randomized clinical trial of laparoscopic total versus anterior 180 degrees fundoplication. Br J Surg. 2005;92:240–3.
17. Baigrie RJ, Cullis SN, Ndhluni AJ, Cariem A. Randomized double-blind trial of laparoscopic Nissen fundoplication versus anterior partial fundoplication. Br J Surg. 2005;92:819–23.
18. Cao Z, Cai W, Qin M, et al. Randomized clinical trial of laparoscopic anterior 180 degrees partial versus 360 degrees Nissen fundoplication: 5-year results. Dis Esophagus. 2012;25:114–20.
19. Raue W, Ordemann J, Jacobi CA, et al. Nissen versus Dor fundoplication for treatment of gastroesophageal reflux disease: a blinded randomized clinical trial. Dig Surg. 2011;28:80–6.
20. Broeders JA, Broeders EA, Watson DI, et al. Objective outcomes 14 years after laparoscopic anterior 180-degree partial versus nissen fundoplication: results from a randomized trial. Ann Surg. 2013;258:233–9.
21. Engstrom C, Lonroth H, Mardani J, Lundell L. An anterior or posterior approach to partial fundoplication? Long-term results of a randomized trial. World J Surg. 2007;31:1221–5; discussion: 1226–7.
22. Watson DI, Jamieson GG, Lally C, et al. Multicenter, prospective, double-blind, randomized trial of laparoscopic nissen vs anterior 90 degrees partial fundoplication. Arch Surg. 2004;139:1160–7.
23. Nijjar RS, Watson DI, Jamieson GG, et al. Five-year follow-up of a multicenter, double-blind randomized clinical trial of laparoscopic Nissen vs anterior 90 degrees partial fundoplication. Arch Surg. 2010;145:552–7.
24. Spence GM, Watson DI, Jamiesion GG, et al. Single center prospective randomized trial of laparoscopic Nissen versus anterior 90 degrees fundoplication. J Gastrointest Surg. 2006;10:698–705.
25. Chisholm JA, Jamieson GG, Lally CJ, et al. The effect of obesity on the outcome of laparoscopic antireflux surgery. J Gastrointest Surg. 2009;13:1064–70.

Chapter 9
Enhancing Clinical Outcomes Through Better Postoperative Management and Follow-Up

Lee L Swanstrom

Acute Postoperative Care

Immediately after surgery, fundoplications enjoy a rather precarious existence. Anesthesia and analgesia-related nausea, in particular, threaten a fresh fundoplication and particularly a recent hiatal hernia repair, with acute disruption or herniation. Patients should have postoperative antiemetics ordered and nurses presented with tiered progressive administration orders and instructions to "treat nausea aggressively." Table 9.1 lists our in-hospital antiemetic regime for fundoplication surgery. Because of the risk of occult post-op vomiting inducing acute herniation, some surgeons have a policy of routine postoperative contrast X-rays on postoperative day 1. Our practice is to obtain gastrografin upper GI studies the morning after the operation for giant hiatal hernia repairs or if the patient had witnessed violent vomiting episodes. If an acute disruption/herniation is detected (Fig. 9.1), we recommend immediate return to the OR for repair. Nausea remains a major threat for fundoplications and endoluminal repairs even after hospital discharge and patients should be given antiemetic prescriptions along with their pain medications on discharge.

Early Postoperative Care and Follow-Up

For the sake of this chapter, we define the early period as the first 3 months after surgery. Patient communication is perhaps the most important during this phase. Patient experience and risks during this time also vary according to the procedure

L.L. Swanstrom, M.D. F.A.C.S., F.A.S.G.E. (✉)
Institut Hospitalo Universitaire—Strasbourg, 1, place de l'Hopital, Strasbourg 67091, France

Division of GI/MIS, The Oregon Clinic—Gastrointestinal & Minimally Invasive Surgery, Portland, OR, USA
e-mail: lswanstrom@gmail.com

© Springer International Publishing Switzerland 2016
R.W. Aye, J.G. Hunter (eds.), *Fundoplication Surgery*,
DOI 10.1007/978-3-319-25094-6_9

123

Table 9.1 Antiemetic
protocols are critical in the
postoperative period

Preoperative on call to OR
• Dexamethasone 10 mg IV
• Ondansetron 4 mg IV
Intraoperative
• Minimize N20
• Minimize narcotics (ketorolac)
Acute recovery
• IV ondansetron 4 mg q 1 h prn
• If no result—phenothiazine IV
• If no result—scopolamine patch
• If no result—sedation (e.g., Lorazepam)
Postoperative hospital care
• IV or sublingual ondansetron prn or scheduled
• If no result—phenothiazine IV
• If no result—scopolamine patch
• If no result—sedation (e.g., Lorazepam)
Post-hospital care
• PRN ondansetron sublingual
• Or phenothiazine suppository
• Instructions to call office if nausea persists

that was performed: for example, pain and dysphagia are patient concerns following laparoscopic Nissen and Hill procedures, less so for Linx and partial fundoplication and not an issue with endoluminal repairs. Regardless, all patients experience "changes" during this period that if not properly explained will frighten, confuse, or even anger the patient and that may—if poorly handled—compromise the outcome of the procedure.

Communication, preferably ahead of time, is the key. At the time of surgery scheduling, we provide the patients with reading material which we have generatede, which describes what they will experience in the hospital, but perhaps more importantly, describes what they will experience after leaving the hospital. As the follow-up after a fundoplication is the most prolonged, we will discuss the key management points for these patients and mention some of the differences between fundoplication, Linx, and endoluminal repairs.

Pain management: Although laparoscopic fundoplication is a minimally invasive approach, it is common for patients to have a moderate amount of postoperative pain. Wound pain is usually minimal, but it is not unusual to have some deep epigastric pain for the first few days to weeks and a third of patients will have some referred left shoulder pain. As this is confusing to patients, they should be warned about it in advance and the concept of referred pain explained. Treatment can be NSAIDS and, if needed, narcotics. Sometimes heat or cold on the shoulder seems to help. The majority of referred shoulder pain resolves within 3 days. Occasionally, it persists for more than a week—this is rare and when it occurs should probably induce a clinic visit since, on very rare occasions, it can indicate a significant prob-

Fig. 9.1 Acute herniation of fundoplication POD 1 following postoperative vomiting

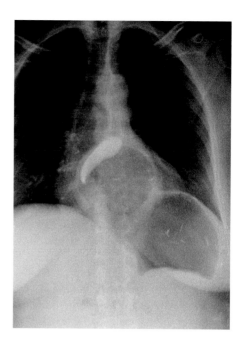

lem (microperforation, wrap herniation, pleural effusion, PE, etc.). Certainly, a workup (chest X-ray, CT scan, or upper endoscopy) is indicated if shoulder pain is not resolved in 3 weeks. Otherwise, patients are given sufficient liquid narcotic to last for 1 week and encouraged to transition to NSAIDs as soon as possible. They should be warned about the side-effects of narcotics, especially nausea and constipation, and instructed to treat these early and aggressively. Patients who present with chest pain due to esophageal spasm should be warned that these spasms can be exacerbated by their surgery. The exacerbation is temporary and usually settles down after a few weeks. Smooth muscle relaxants may help this situation.

Wound care: Laparoscopic wounds need little care, but patients should be informed regarding when to remove dressings and what to look for regarding complications such as infections.

Activity: In general, aside from eating, antireflux patients need little activity restriction aside from warnings about doing things while taking narcotics. The exception is large hiatal hernia repairs, which, as with most tensioned hernia repairs, commonly occasion some restriction and graduated return to activity. How much and how long varies widely across practices, but should be spelled out very concretely and in writing to the patient. For giant hiatal hernia repairs, we generally recommend 4–6 weeks of minimal lifting (<15 lbs) and avoidance of strenuous activities.

Nausea: Retching and vomiting is probably the greatest stressor for antireflux surgeries of all types. We always send patients home with nausea medication (sublingual ondansetron or promethazine suppositories) and give explicit instructions to treat nausea early and aggressively. In fact, we tell patients to try to avoid vomiting for life and encourage them to keep some antiemetic medication of prescription close at hand for cases of food poisoning, gastroenteritis, etc.

Eating: Little causes more confusion and stress on antireflux patients than postoperative diet instructions. Once again, there is tremendous variation between practitioners, though most will advise an altered diet for at least a period of time after a fundoplication. It's distressing for the patient and family to have food sticking and can lead to retching which may harm the repair. An exception to this is the instructions post-Linx which encourage a solid diet as soon as possible in order to "exercise" the magnetic links and minimize encapsulation. Patients should be cautioned beforehand, however, that this does not mean they won't have dysphagia. In fact, Linx is rather dysphagiagenic in the early months.

For fundoplications, we routinely instruct patients to maintain a pureed diet, including liquid or crushed medications, for the first 2 weeks, and then slowly advance to a regular diet, saving breads, meats, and raw vegetables to the last. We find that it is imperative to spell this out explicitly in the written instructions given to the patient—preferably before the operation. Ideally you should describe the exact texture of the diet you order in graphic detail, and even better, provide sample recipes for the patient. The more detailed and explicit your instructions, the fewer late phone calls and ER visits one will deal with.

Dysphagia: Patients should be forewarned about postoperative dysphagia. Early teaching that this is normal and indicates that their physiologic reflux barrier is working will prevent panic and anguished calls in the early recovery phase. In fact, we once studied those patients who *didn't* have post-op dysphagia after a Nissen fundoplication to make sure their long-term outcomes weren't lessened—they weren't [1].

There are special issues to be aware of with regard to dysphagia. The first as mentioned is the Linx. As patients are told to eat solids from the beginning, they almost all notice some dysphagia. They must be warned, however, that the dysphagia gets worse several weeks after surgery. This is presumably due to the acute phase of the peri-Linx scar tissue and resolves as the scar remodels and softens. For laparoscopic fundoplications, while dysphagia post-op is normal, it should resolve within weeks to months after the procedure. We define abnormal postoperative dysphagia as inability to eat solids, (but not necessarily bread and meat), more than 3 weeks after surgery.

Abnormal dysphagia post-fundoplication can be categorized as either persistent dysphagia or new onset. Persistent dysphagia is difficulty swallowing immediately after surgery, which doesn't improve in the early follow-up. It may be due to abnormally prolonged edema, but may also be due to an intrinsic motility disorder, an overly tight or improper fundoplication, or an anatomic problem like wrap herniation. After 3 weeks, a comprehensive evaluation is indicated to rule out any underlying problems such as these as they probably won't get better on their own. If no underlying physiology or anatomic problems are found, an endoscopy with empiric dilatation is often helpful. If the patient could initially swallow but then develops dysphagia, it is typically due to either early wrap herniation or an inflammation caused by food impaction or an infection such as esophageal candidiasis. A diagnostic upper endoscopy is almost always indicated and a gentle dilation should resolve the issue (Fig. 9.2).

Fig. 9.2 Suspect candida (or other) esophagitis if the patient presents with acute postoperative dysphagia after a period of normal swallowing

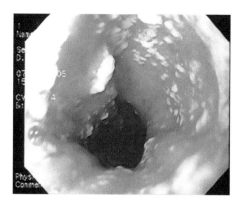

Gas: Bloating and flatulence are experienced by the majority of fundoplication patients and are often a source of bitterness and a perception of a reduced quality of life (QOL), which is often baffling to surgeons [2]. In fact, gas-related complaints are probably the major reason that Nissen is considered "patient unfriendly." No doubt, this is also the major reason patients opt for alternative treatments like Linx and endoluminal ARS. Ironically, objective analysis has confirmed that GERD patients preoperatively are "gassy" and in fact bloating and belching are usually improved post-fundoplication, although flatulence may not be [3]. Early difficulty belching and decreased gastric capacity and compliance account for the increased negative perception of gas post-fundoplication. In general, the earlier and better patients can belch post-fundoplication, the better the gas symptoms are, which is why some surgeons prefer a partial fundoplication like the Toupet which has been shown to have a better "belch profile" if you will [4]. Once again, aggressive education is important. Before surgery, the surgeon should warn the patient about a "gassy period" after surgery and explain the physiology behind aerophagia and GERD. Patients should be given written postoperative instructions also explaining gas during the early/intermediate post-op period and offering explicit instructions to ameliorate the symptoms. This should include avoidance of carbonated beverages, gas-forming foods, chewing gum, drinking too fast, drinking with a straw, etc. Patients should be encouraged to take simethicone-containing medications on a routine basis. Most of all, they should be reassured that as edema reduces and gastric accommodation improves, this symptom will almost always get better (or they will adjust to it). There are occasional patients who feel crippled by gas-related symptoms even after 6 months to a year. If they can't belch, it is worth performing an EGD to check for evidence of delayed gastric emptying or gastric pathology and to perform an empiric dilatation (56–60 Fr). Continued problems may warrant a radionucleide gastric emptying exam, attempts at gut sterilization, or referral to a gastroenterologist or naturopath or a speech therapist for coaching against aerophagia. On very rare occasions, gas complaints have led to a conversion of a Nissen to a partial wrap or even total reversal of the procedure.

Heartburn: Ninety-seven percent of patients have resolution of their heartburn in the early postoperative period [5]. The 3 % who don't are truly problematic. They should be encouraged to wait as long as possible before evaluation or treatment—ideally even 6 months. Oral antacids, GI cocktail, or restarting PPI's are certainly OK. If symptoms prove persistent, an exhaustive retesting should be performed, including endoscopy with biopsy to rule out inflammatory or infectious causes (or a failed fundoplication) and 24 h impedance pH testing to prove or disprove gastroesophageal reflux and to look for stasis from a too-tight wrap. Hopefully, you will have a preoperative study to compare to. Very often in this small patient subset, no explanation is found, any reflux has been fixed, and there is little to offer.

Late Follow-Up

Late follow-up, 3 months to a year for the sake of this chapter, is important as well. It is during this period that most postoperative side effects should have resolved and the patient achieved homeostasis. This is also the period where they will have forgotten all their instructions and lost their postoperative care instruction manual and may have regressed to bad habits, vomiting, carbonated beverages, overeating etc. We routinely see patients at 6 months and a year to touch bases, answer questions, and repeat their coaching. We also perform comprehensive postoperative testing to objectively confirm the integrity of their repair. It is our belief that at a minimum, an EGD to assess the wrap and a 24 h pH test should be performed between 6 and 12 months. We and others have shown that postoperative symptoms have a poor correlation with GERD post-fundoplication [6, 7]. In our experience, 50 % of patients having heartburn complaints postoperatively have absolutely no reflux on pH testing. Conversely, 13 % of patients with no heartburn have pathologic reflux and are probably best treated with acid suppression to prevent GERD-related complications.

We also encourage a repeat manometry to look for resolution of motility issues, onset of new motility issues, or a problem with the LES. Certainly, a manometry is indicated if the patient has dysphagia symptoms during this period.

Long-Term Follow-Up

Antireflux surgery of any variety is a mechanical intervention in a physiologic process. Without some fundamental change in the patient's behaviors—and possibly their genetics—almost all of these mechanical fixes would eventually fail. The exception, perhaps, is the Linx procedure, which theoretically, unless it erodes, will provide the same barrier in 1000 years. Late failure of fundoplications is both difficult to predict and difficult to define. We usually warn patients that laparoscopic antireflux procedures are not a definitive cure and will fail at around 1 % per year [8]. This makes it reasonable to encourage long-term follow-up for patients—interesting both from an academic and quality assurance basis and from a desire to pick up late-term problems early in patients. In North

America, due to cost concerns, routine follow-up imaging or diagnostic studies are probably not feasible, unless the patient has Barretts esophagus and meets society-derived screening criteria. None-the-less, much information can be gained by administering a structured symptom evaluation over the long-term and we routinely encourage our patients to come back every 2–3 years to touch bases. If the patient does present with some new onset symptoms, an aggressive work up is indicated before simply putting them on a PPI and dismissing them: UGI X-ray for dysphagia or pain, EGD and pH study for recurrent heartburn, etc.

Surveillance Data Collection and Tools

As has been stressed throughout this chapter, consistent, thorough, and long-term follow-up is critical to ensure the best outcomes following antireflux surgery. Objective data is critical both to determine the optimal surgery and to truly understand what the *mechanical* effect of the surgery on the disease is. None-the-less, objective information must always be tied to the patient's perception of their disease and its impact on their QOL. We have therefore always felt that it is absolutely imperative to assess the patient's perception of their disease and its impact on their life throughout their care. We feel the best way to accomplish this is to administer a structured and quantified symptom evaluation questionnaire when the patient is first seen and every time subsequently. Also, as symptoms are only important in so far as they impact the patient's life, it doesn't hurt to also administer and track QOL—though processing and tracking this type of data requires more of a research infrastructure embedded in one's clinical practice. For the latter, there are numerous validated QOL surveys. These come in 2 basic classes: either a general lifestyle impact (e.g., SF-36) or a "disease specific" format (e.g., GERD-HQOL) [9, 10]. These self-administered questionnaires are subsequently scored and compared to population norms—usually by an external agent (for a price).

Perhaps even more important for patient education and internal evaluation are symptom assessment forms. There are fewer commercially available and validated examples of these, at least in a global form, though aspects (e.g., dysphagia or GERD symptoms) do exist [11, 12]. We have administered basically the same symptom assessment form since 1991. It questions the patient on primary symptom, current medication use, effectiveness of medication, symptom time-frame, previous interventions, and then includes a 4-point Likert scale-based assessment of symptoms—heartburn, regurgitation, dysphagia, chest pain, gas symptoms, respiratory symptoms (cough, globus, etc.). Responses to this are elicited and recorded by the provider as opposed to a self-reported format. Also important is the assessment of secondary symptoms—abdominal pain, nausea, cough, diarrhea, flatulence, etc.—items that to surgeons often seem peripheral or "psychological" but which may play a central role in the satisfaction of the patient with the proposed procedure.

It is important that responses to the symptom assessment form are saved in a hierarchical format that allows the practitioner to track long-term changes and—

importantly—share these with the patient. This can be in a simple electronic spread-sheet—if it is for basic tracking and comparisons—or a more sophisticated database that allows queries, which is especially useful if one performs outcomes research. Of course the later sort of prospective research database requires institutional ethical approval and patient consent, but, in return, this obviates IRB approval for individual studies based on the patient's records. It can't be stressed enough how often the ability to present to the patient how their own report of their current condition compares to how they reported their initial condition before intervention alters their self-perception and satisfaction with the procedure. For the practitioner, such longitudinal and consistent data recording is both an important research tool, but also a way to honestly assess one's outcomes—potentially altering one's approach to the next patient to improve objective and subjective outcomes.

Conclusion

The key to optimizing operative outcomes in reflux surgery can be distilled into three precepts: Educate the patient proactively, obsessively follow the patient with quantifiable data collection tools and, dispassionately study this gathered information and be willing to change your practice based on the results. A patient who is told what to expect, and *why*, will be happier and less of a management problem. The ability to compare where the patient started from, what you did based on your understanding of their problem at the time, and objective and subjective outcomes over time are the most powerful tools a surgeon has to improve one's treatment philosophy and practice.

References

1. Makris KI, Cassera MA, Kastenmeier AS, Dunst CM, Swanström LL. Postoperative dysphagia is not predictive of long-term failure after laparoscopic antireflux surgery. Surg Endosc. 2011;26(2):451–7.
2. Swanstrom LL, Wayne R. Spectrum of gastrointestinal symptoms after laparoscopic fundoplication. Am J Surg. 1994;167(5):538–41.
3. Rantanen T, Kiljander T, Salminen P, Ranta A, Oksala N, Kellokumpu I. Reflux symptoms and side effects among patients with gastroesophageal reflux disease at baseline, during treatment with PPIs, and after Nissen fundoplication. World J Surg. 2013;37(6):1291–6. doi:10.1007/s00268-013-1979-8.
4. Broeders JA, Bredenoord AJ, Hazebroek EJ, Broeders IA, Gooszen HG, Smout AJ. Reflux and belching after 270 degree versus 360 degree laparoscopic posterior fundoplication. Ann Surg. 2012;255(1):59–65.
5. Lundell L. Surgical therapy of gastro-oesophageal reflux disease. Best Pract Res Clin Gastroenterol. 2010;24(6):947–59.
6. Khajanchee YS, O'Rourke RW, Lockhart BA, Patterson EJ, Hansen PD, Swanstrom LL. Postoperative Symptoms and failure following antireflux surgery. Arch Surg. 2002;137(9):1008–14.

7. Chan K, Liu G, Miller L, Ma C, Xu W, Schlachta CM, Darling G. Lack of correlation between a self-administered subjective GERD questionnaire and pathologic GERD diagnosed by 24-h esophageal pH monitoring. J Gastrointest Surg. 2010;14(3):427–36.
8. Robinson B, Dunst CM, Cassera MA, Reavis KM, Sharata A, Swanström LL. 20 years later: laparoscopic fundoplication durability. Surg Endosc. 2015;29(9):2520–4.
9. Kaji M, Fujiwara Y, Shiba M, Kohata Y, Yamagami H, Tanigawa T, Watanabe K, Watanabe T, Tominaga K, Arakawa T. Prevalence of overlaps between GERD, FD and IBS and impact on health-related quality of life. J Gastroenterol Hepatol. 2010;25(6):1151–6.
10. Chan Y, Ching JY, Cheung CM, Tsoi KK, Polder-Verkiel S, Pang SH, Quan WL, Kee KM, Chan FK, Sung JJ, Wu JC. Development and validation of a disease-specific quality of life questionnaire for gastro-oesophageal reflux disease: the GERD-QOL questionnaire. Aliment Pharmacol Ther. 2010;31(3):452–60.
11. Armstrong D, Mönnikes H, Bardhan KD, Stanghellini V. The construction of a new evaluative GERD questionnaire—methods and state of the art. Digestion. 2007;75 Suppl 1:17–24.
12. Kwiatek MA, Kiebles JL, Taft TH, Pandolfino JE, Bové MJ, Kahrilas PJ, Keefer L. Esophageal symptoms questionnaire for the assessment of dysphagia, globus, and reflux symptoms: initial development and validation. Dis Esophagus. 2011;24(8):550–9.

Chapter 10
How to Build the Trust of Your Referring Physicians

Stuart Jon Spechler

Very few (if any) peer-reviewed publications have dealt specifically with the issue of how surgeons might build trust in the physicians who refer patients to them for antireflux surgery. Consequently, my comments in this chapter are based largely on my personal experience and opinion. I do feel that my decades of experience as a researcher and a practicing gastroenterologist with a specific interest in gastro-esophageal reflux disease (GERD) have given me some perspective on this issue that others might find useful. Nevertheless, the reader should be cautioned that much of this chapter is more "eminence-based" than evidence-based.

Of course, a surgeon's experience, technical skills, and medical judgment are key issues that a physician considers when making any surgical referral. There is also much truth to the old adage that the three pillars of a successful medical or surgical practice are the doctor's three A's—Availability, Affability, and Ability (perhaps in that order). *However, in my opinion, the most important consideration regarding trust when referring a patient for antireflux surgery is the surgeon's honesty about the operation.* This includes honesty in discussing the risks and benefits of alternative treatment options, in realistically appraising the operation's anticipated benefits and in clearly presenting the potential complications of fundoplication. Many patients with GERD, especially those with Barrett's esophagus, are very concerned about their risk of developing esophageal adenocarcinoma. *When referring such patients, a physician will develop trust in a surgeon who does not exaggerate the risk of this cancer for patients with GERD, and who does not present fundoplication*

S.J. Spechler, M.D. (✉)
Department of Medicine, Esophageal Diseases Center, VA North Texas Healthcare System, University of Texas Southwestern Medical Center, Dallas, TX, USA

Division of Gastroenterology and Hepatology (111B1), Dallas VA Medical Center, 4500 South Lancaster Road, Dallas, TX 75216, USA
e-mail: sjspechler@aol.com

© Springer International Publishing Switzerland 2016
R.W. Aye, J.G. Hunter (eds.), *Fundoplication Surgery*,
DOI 10.1007/978-3-319-25094-6_10

133

as clearly superior to medical therapy for cancer prevention (which it is not). Such tactics are often construed, appropriately or not, as attempts to frighten a patient into an operation on false pretenses, tactics that are not likely to instill trust.

Medical vs. Surgical Therapy for GERD

When choosing between medical and surgical treatments for GERD, it is important to appreciate that both of these treatments generally will do exactly what they were designed to do. The modern medical therapy for GERD focuses almost exclusively on the control of gastric acid production with antisecretory medications like proton pump inhibitors (PPIs) [1]. The PPIs were designed to inhibit gastric acid production and, therefore, they decrease acid reflux. Consequently, they usually provide excellent relief for symptoms caused by acid reflux. However, the PPIs do not prevent the reflux of nonacidic material, and they will not relieve symptoms or prevent complications caused by nonacidic reflux. Fundoplication was designed to create a barrier to the reflux of all gastric material, acidic and nonacidic. Consequently, fundoplication usually provides excellent relief for symptoms caused by reflux but, of course, fundoplication will not relieve symptoms that are not caused by reflux. *As obvious as this assertion might seem, the major problem that I have seen with fundoplication over the years is when it is used in an attempt to treat symptoms that are not caused by reflux. That is when antireflux surgery is doomed to fail.*

PPIs were not designed to correct the defective antireflux mechanisms that underlie the development of GERD and, consequently, acid reflux usually returns shortly after PPIs are stopped. Indeed, for patients who have severe GERD complicated by erosive reflux esophagitis, a number of studies have shown that erosive esophagitis redevelops in the large majority of cases when PPI therapy is discontinued [2]. Consequently, patients with erosive esophagitis essentially have only two choices for GERD control—lifelong PPI therapy or antireflux surgery.

The PPIs are among the safest classes of medications used by gastroenterologists, and the most common PPI side effects are minor (e.g., headache, diarrhea, constipation, abdominal discomfort) and rarely are a cause for major clinical concern. However, there are a number of more serious risks that have been proposed for chronic PPI therapy [3]. These can be divided into five general categories: (1) Concern that, by increasing serum gastrin levels and enabling bacteria to colonize the stomach, PPIs might increase the risk for developing colon cancer, gastric cancer, and cancer in Barrett's esophagus, (2) Concern that, by decreasing gastric acid production, PPIs might increase the risk of developing a variety of infections such as community-acquired pneumonia, enteric infections, and *C. difficile* colitis, (3) Concern that PPI effects on vitamin and mineral metabolism might cause deficiencies, including low serum vitamin B12 and magnesium levels, and might result in bone fractures, (4) Concerns regarding PPI effects on the metabolism of other drugs such as clopidogrel and methotrexate, and (5) A number of proposed miscellaneous side effects such as interstitial nephritis, microscopic colitis, celiac disease, and cardiovascular events in patients with acute coronary syndrome.

Most of these "risks" are far more theoretical than real. For example, there are no convincing data that PPIs increase the risk for any human malignancy. Nevertheless, these potential side effects have received much attention in the medical and lay press, and physicians and patients alike should be concerned about the potential consequences of chronic PPI therapy.

I feel that it is always an appropriate and good medical practice to discuss these potential PPI risks with GERD patients who face a lifetime of treatment with these medications. No medical treatment is without risks, and it is the physician's job to convey that point to patients. *Nevertheless, a surgeon who emphasizes or exaggerates the largely theoretical concerns regarding PPIs in order to promote antireflux surgery will promptly lose the trust of the referring physician.* The association of PPIs with most of these proposed side effects is dubious and, even if real, the increase in the frequency of these adverse events (e.g., hip fractures), above those of age- and sex-matched patients who do not take PPIs, is relatively small. Furthermore, a number of studies have documented that many, if not most, patients who have antireflux surgery will be prescribed PPI therapy at some point *after* the operation [4, 5]. Although a large proportion of these PPI prescriptions might be inappropriate, they are prescribed anyway and *patients should not be promised that fundoplication will permanently eliminate PPI therapy and its attendant risks.* Such a promise is likely to be broken, and broken promises are a good way to destroy trust.

I assume that most readers of this chapter are surgeons who are well aware that fundoplication can have considerable adverse outcomes [6], and I will not belabor this point. Suffice it to say that there are serious operative complications of fundoplication including esophageal perforation, bleeding, splenic injury and, rarely, death. Fundoplication also can have not-so-rare, long-term side effects like dysphagia, gas-bloat syndrome, delayed gastric emptying, and diarrhea, and these problems occasionally can be very difficult to manage and very detrimental to quality of life. The surgeon should also consider that, in the large majority of cases, GERD is a benign condition that responds well to medical therapy. For patients who have typical GERD symptoms that are well-controlled by medications, and who are satisfied with that therapy, it is difficult to justify an invasive procedure like fundoplication that can have troublesome, difficult to manage, and even fatal side effects.

It is possible to make some excellent theoretical arguments about why fundoplication should be better than medical therapy for preventing GERD complications such as esophageal strictures and adenocarcinoma. Medical therapy targets gastric acid almost exclusively, but acid is not the only potentially harmful agent in gastric juice. Refluxed bile acids might contribute to esophageal injury and carcinogenesis, and an effective antireflux operation is a barrier to the reflux of all noxious gastric material, including bile acids. Some relatively small, observational studies have suggested that surgically treated patients with Barrett's esophagus develop less dysplasia and cancer than their medically treated counterparts. However, high-quality studies (including two randomized trials [1, 7], two meta-analyses [8, 9], and three studies that used very large databases [10–12]) have found no significant difference in cancer incidence between medically and surgically treated GERD patients. Both medical and surgical GERD therapies appear to protect against GERD complications, including esophageal adenocarcinoma, but fundoplication should not be recommended solely with the rationale that it provides better protection than medical therapy. *A surgeon who proposes fundoplication to patients who are happy with their medical therapy on the grounds that fundoplication is better for preventing GERD complications should not garner the trust of referring physicians.*

PPI-Refractory GERD

An interesting study by Campos et al. evaluated the predictors of successful outcome for 199 consecutive patients who had laparoscopic Nissen fundoplication, and who were followed for a median of 15 months [13]. The operation had a good or excellent outcome in 87 % of study patients, and a fair or poor outcome in 13 %. *By multivariate analysis, the three factors that predicted a successful surgical outcome were abnormal acid reflux documented by 24-h pH monitoring, a typical primary GERD symptom (e.g., heartburn, regurgitation), and a clinical response to acid suppression. Thus, the patients who did best with surgery were the patients with typical GERD that responded well to medical therapy.* In my opinion, the reason that the three factors identified by this study worked so well to predict the outcome of surgery was because these factors identify patients who clearly have GERD symptoms due to acid reflux. It is not surprising that PPIs and antireflux surgery both work well in those patients, because both of these therapies are excellent for controlling acid reflux. However, patients with typical GERD symptoms that respond well to PPI therapy infrequently are referred for an antireflux operation.

PPIs heal reflux esophagitis in the large majority of cases, but PPIs fail to completely eliminate symptoms attributed to GERD in up to 40 % of patients [14]. That is the group most frequently referred for antireflux operations. Although the PPIs are far from perfect in eliminating GERD symptoms, *failure to respond to PPIs nevertheless is a red flag that should alert the astute clinician that GERD might not be the cause of symptoms.* Patients with PPI-refractory GERD will benefit from antireflux surgery only if their refractory "GERD symptoms" really are due to GERD. Unfortunately, many (if not most) patients thought to have PPI-refractory GERD do not have GERD as the cause of their refractory symptoms. Often, these refractory symptoms are not the typical GERD symptoms of heartburn and regurgitation, but atypical symptoms like chest pain, hoarseness, and chronic cough. Although GERD frequently is blamed for these atypical symptoms, that diagnosis often is mistaken and GERD is not the cause of the atypical symptoms in many cases. Thus, before proceeding with an operation to correct GERD, it is critical for the surgeon to establish that GERD is in fact the cause of symptoms. The most technically exquisite antireflux operation will not benefit a patient whose symptoms are not due to GERD. The surgeon who operates without first ensuring that GERD is indeed the cause of symptoms will have frequent failures, which will destroy the trust of the referring physician.

There are at least six reasons why "GERD symptoms" might persist during PPI therapy: [15] (1) Abnormal acid reflux persists despite PPI treatment. (2) Acid reflux has normalized with PPIs, but even the "normal" amounts of acid reflux cause symptoms; these first two conditions can be identified by esophageal pH monitoring while the patient remains on PPI therapy. (3) The reflux of nonacidic material causes symptoms; this condition can be identified by multichannel intraluminal impedance (MII) monitoring, but available studies on the utility of the test for this purpose are limited and an expert group (the Esophageal Diagnostic Advisory Panel) recently concluded that there are insufficient data to justify the use of MII data alone as the basis for recommending antireflux surgery (5). (4) Symptoms are caused by an esophageal disorder other than GERD (e.g., eosinophilic esophagitis, achalasia); these disorders can be identified by endoscopy and esophageal manometry. (5) Symptoms are caused by an extra-esophageal disorder (e.g., heart disease, biliary tract disease); these disorders can be identified with appropriate tests on an individual basis depending on the clinical situation. (6) Symptoms are functional (i.e., not due to GERD or any other histopathology-based disorder, esophageal or extra-esophageal). The surgeon who considers and explores these possibilities before embarking on an antireflux operation for a patient with "PPI-refractory GERD symptoms" should earn the trust of the referring physician.

The Esophageal Diagnostic Advisory Panel has published a consensus statement on what diagnostic tests they feel are necessary to establish the presence and severity of GERD in patients being considered for antireflux surgery [16]. They first recommended endoscopy, noting that the demonstration of severe reflux esophagitis (Los Angeles grade C or D) or long-segment Barrett's esophagus (≥3 cm Barrett's metaplasia) firmly establishes a diagnosis of GERD. They also recommended a barium esophagram to define anatomic features such as hiatal hernia size and type that might be important for surgical planning. Esophageal manometry was recommended both to rule out achalasia (which can have symptoms of heartburn, regurgitation, and dysphagia that can be confused with GERD) and to "tailor" the type of fundoplication to be performed (avoiding tight wraps for patients with poor motility). Regarding esophageal pH monitoring, the experts felt that this could be omitted when endoscopy shows severe reflux esophagitis or long-segment Barrett's esophagus, but should be performed routinely (off acid suppression) for patients who have only mild (Los Angeles grade A or B) or no erosive esophagitis, and for patients with only short-segment or no Barrett's esophagus. Finally, for patients refractory to PPIs, the experts suggested pH testing (on acid suppression) with or without multichannel intraluminal impedance monitoring. Again, these recommendations emphasize the need to establish firmly that the patient has GERD and that the patient's symptoms are a result of GERD. Adherence to these guidelines will maximize the chance for surgical success, which will go a long way in building trust in the referring physician.

Follow-Up

One final area worthy of mention in regard to building the trust of the referring physician is that of patients' follow-up. The referring physician appreciates a surgeon who becomes a partner in the care of the patient. The surgeon who merely performs the operation and immediate postoperative follow-up, and then declares the job done, leaving the referring physician to manage operative side effects and other recovery issues is not likely to receive many repeat referrals. Both the referring physician and the patient will appreciate the surgeon who takes responsibility for postoperative issues, and who assumes an active role as a partner in long-term patient care.

Conclusion

A referring physician will learn to trust a surgeon who has excellent outcomes, and there is no question that many patients and their physicians are delighted with the outcome of antireflux surgery. For the antireflux surgeon, a major step in achieving excellent outcomes is to ensure that the symptoms that prompted the referral for fundoplication indeed are due to GERD. This can be accomplished by adherence to the diagnostic approach outlined above. *When it is clear that the troublesome symptoms are due to reflux that can be corrected by fundoplication, the surgeon should be completely straightforward with the patient in appraising the operation's anticipated benefits and in clearly presenting the potential complications of fundoplication. The surgeon should not exaggerate the risk of esophageal adenocarcinoma or other complications of GERD, which can be construed as an attempt to frighten a patient into having an antireflux operation. Since there are no convincing data that such operations are superior to medical therapy for preventing GERD complications, the surgeon also should not exaggerate the degree of protection from GERD complications afforded by fundoplication.* In my opinion, the primary goal of an antireflux operation is to correct symptoms not adequately addressed by medical therapy. Surgeons who have earned my trust over the years are those that have adhered to the approach outlined above.

References

1. Katz PO, Gerson LB, Vela MF. Guidelines for the diagnosis and management of gastroesophageal reflux disease. Am J Gastroenterol. 2013;108:308–28.
2. Dent J, Hetzel DJ, MacKinnon MA, Reed WD, Narielvala FM. Evaluation of omeprazole in reflux oesophagitis. Scand J Gastroenterol Suppl. 1989;166:76–82.
3. Johnson DA, Oldfield IV EC. Reported side effects and complications of long-term proton pump inhibitor use: dissecting the evidence. Clin Gastroenterol Hepatol. 2013;11:458–64.
4. Spechler SJ, Lee E, Ahnen D, Goyal RK, Hirano I, Ramirez F, Raufman JP, Sampliner R, Schnell T, Sontag S, Vlahcevic ZR, Young R, Williford W. Long-term outcome of medical and surgical treatments for gastroesophageal reflux disease. Follow-up of a randomized controlled trial. JAMA. 2001;285:2331–8.
5. Lundell L, Miettinen P, Myrvold HE, Hatlebakk JG, Wallin L, Engström C, Julkunen R, Montgomery M, Malm A, Lind T, Walan A, Nordic GERD Study Group. Comparison of outcomes twelve years after antireflux surgery or omeprazole maintenance therapy for reflux esophagitis. Clin Gastroenterol Hepatol. 2009;7:1292–8.
6. Spechler SJ. The management of patients who have "failed" antireflux surgery. Am J Gastroenterol. 2004;99:552–61.

7. Parrilla P, Martínez de Haro LF, Ortiz A, Munitiz V, Molina J, Bermejo J, Canteras M. Long-term results of a randomized prospective study comparing medical and surgical treatment of Barrett's esophagus. Ann Surg. 2003;237:291–8.
8. Corey KE, Schmitz SM, Shaheen NJ. Does a surgical antireflux procedure decrease the incidence of esophageal adenocarcinoma in Barrett's esophagus? A meta-analysis. Am J Gastroenterol. 2003;98:2390–4.
9. Chang EY, Morris CD, Seltman AK, O'Rourke RW, Chan BK, Hunter JG, Jobe BA. The effect of antireflux surgery on esophageal carcinogenesis in patients with Barrett esophagus: a systematic review. Ann Surg. 2007;246:11–21.
10. Ye W, Chow WH, Lagergren J, Yin L, Nyrén O. Risk of adenocarcinomas of the esophagus and gastric cardia in patients with gastroesophageal reflux diseases and after antireflux surgery. Gastroenterology. 2001;121:1286–93.
11. Tran T, Spechler SJ, El-Serag HB. Fundoplication and the risk of cancer in gastroesophageal reflux disease: a veterans affairs cohort study. Am J Gastroenterol. 2005;100:1002–8.
12. Lagergren J, Ye W, Lagergren P, Lu Y. The risk of esophageal adenocarcinoma after antireflux surgery. Gastroenterology. 2010;138:1297–301.
13. Campos GM, Peters JH, DeMeester TR, Oberg S, Crookes PF, Tan S, DeMeester SR, Hagen JA, Bremner CG. Multivariate analysis of factors predicting outcome after laparoscopic Nissen fundoplication. J Gastrointest Surg. 1999;3:292–300.
14. Castell DO, Kahrilas PJ, Richter JE, Vakil NB, Johnson DA, Zuckerman S, Skammer W, Levine JG. Esomeprazole (40 mg) compared with lansoprazole (30 mg) in the treatment of erosive esophagitis. Am J Gastroenterol. 2002;97:575–83.
15. Spechler SJ. Surgery for gastroesophageal reflux disease: esophageal impedance to progress? Clin Gastroenterol Hepatol. 2009;7:1264–5.
16. Jobe BA, Richter JE, Hoppo T, Peters JH, Bell R, Dengler WC, DeVault K, Fass R, Gyawali CP, Kahrilas PJ, Lacy BE, Pandolfino JE, Patti MG, Swanstrom LL, Kurian AA, Vela MF, Vaezi M, DeMeester TR. Preoperative diagnostic workup before antireflux surgery: an evidence and experience-based consensus of the Esophageal Diagnostic Advisory Panel. J Am Coll Surg. 2013;217:586–97.

Chapter 11
Diagnosis and Management of Gastroesophageal Reflux Disease in Pediatric Patients

Gretchen Purcell Jackson

Gastroesophageal Reflux Disease in Infants and Children

Gastroesophageal reflux (GER) is defined as passage of gastric contents into the esophagus with or without vomiting, and it is a normal physiological process in both children and adults. In contrast, gastroesophageal reflux disease (GERD) is GER that produces significant symptoms or complications, such as recurrent vomiting or aspiration pneumonia [1]. GER is present in over two thirds of healthy infants and often manifests as baby "spit ups." Over half of healthy infants regurgitate daily from physiological GER [2].

The symptoms and complications that define GERD vary with the age of the patient, are relatively non-specific, and can be classified as esophageal or extraesophageal. In infants, common esophageal GERD manifestations include vomiting and poor weight gain. While infants cannot report retrosternal chest pain associated with reflux, they may demonstrate symptoms such as irritability, arching of the back, feeding refusal, and sleep disruptions. Extraesophageal findings seen with GERD in infants include coughing, choking, wheezing, and other upper respiratory symptoms. Both GER and GERD are extremely common in infants, and distinguishing these entities is critical in determining whether treatment is warranted. The incidence of GERD peaks at approximately 50 % at 4 months, but falls to 5–10 % by 1 year of age. Most GER, GERD, and the associated symptoms seen in infancy will resolve by the age of 12–18 months, so the severity of the symptoms or complications must be weighed carefully against the risks of invasive diagnostic or therapeutic procedures in the first year of life [2].

G.P. Jackson, M.D., Ph.D. (✉)
Department of Pediatric Surgery, Monroe Carell Jr. Children's Hospital at Vanderbilt,
Doctor's Office Tower Suite 7100, 2200 Children's Way, Nashville, TN 37232, USA
e-mail: gretchen.jackson@vanderbilt.edu

© Springer International Publishing Switzerland 2016
R.W. Aye, J.G. Hunter (eds.), *Fundoplication Surgery*,
DOI 10.1007/978-3-319-25094-6_11

Children and adolescents may present with classic adult esophageal symptoms of GERD including heartburn, dysphagia, and sour burps, as well as the findings more characteristic of pediatric GERD such as vomiting, feeding aversion, poor weight gain, and even malnutrition in severe cases. Extraesophageal manifestations of GERD in this population can include chronic cough, hoarseness, asthma, recurrent pneumonia, and dental erosions [2]. Unfortunately, neither individual symptoms nor constellations of symptoms accurately predict GERD or response to treatment in infants and young children [1]. Once able to talk, children can communicate symptoms of GERD-associated pain, but their reports are not thought to be reliable for diagnosis until the ages of 8–12 years [3–6]. Although limited in infancy and early childhood, a thorough history and physical examination may be adequate to diagnose GERD in the adolescent patient with typical symptoms [1].

Several pediatric populations have a high risk of GERD and its complications, which may be difficult to diagnose due to the comorbid illnesses. Conditions associated with pediatric GERD include prematurity, neurological impairment, chronic respiratory disease, obesity, esophageal atresia and other congenital esophageal disorders, and a history of lung transplantation or repaired achalasia. For these patients, a high index of suspicion and low threshold for screening for GERD are warranted, especially when considering gastrostomy tube placement for long-term enteral access [1, 2].

Diagnosis

Intraluminal esophageal pH monitoring and multiple intraluminal impedance (MII)monitoring are the primary studies used to establish definitely a diagnosis of GERD in pediatric patients [7–9]. Intraluminal pH monitoring quantifies the duration and frequency of acid exposure within the esophagus over time. MII monitoring evaluates changes in electrical impedance between a series of electrodes positioned along an esophageal catheter. MII can provide detailed information about the velocity and direction of movements of air, fluids, and solids within the esophagus. Electrodes to measure pH can be combined with MII electrodes on the same esophageal catheter to allow the measurement of acidity of refluxed material. Combined pH and MII monitoring is considered the gold standard test to diagnose GERD, to correlate symptoms with both acidic and nonacidic reflux events, and to evaluate responses to GERD therapy in children [7–9].

Several additional studies may be indicated in infants and children to rule out confounding or alternative diagnoses [1, 2]. For newborns with progressive and nonbilious vomiting, an ultrasound study should be done to rule out hypertrophic pyloric stenosis. Pyloric stenosis generally presents at 42–48 weeks' postconceptual age and is treated with surgical pyloromyotomy [10, 11]. In infants or young children with suspected GERD, an upper gastrointestinal contrast study is usually performed to evaluate for malrotation or other congenital anatomic abnormalities, such as a duodenal web. The upper gastrointestinal contrast study is not useful for diagnosing pathological reflux, but it may identify malrotation in up to 4 % of children with symptoms of reflux [12]. Malrotation occurs in 1 of 500 live births, often with other congenital abnormalities, and it can cause or exacerbate GERD with duodenal bands or midgut volvulus producing partial or intermittent proximal obstruction. If malrotation is identified in a child with GERD, most pediatric surgeons recommend a Ladd procedure as first-line therapy [13]. The Ladd procedure involves division of any adhesive bands (i.e., Ladd's bands) across the duodenum and the base of the mesentery to address duodenal obstruction and reduce the risk of midgut volvulus. A prophylactic appendectomy is usually performed as the appendix is not located in the right lower quadrant of the abdomen in individuals with malrotation, making the presentation of appendicitis atypical [14]. The child with malrotation and GERD should be reevaluated for reflux after recovery from the Ladd's procedure. In many patients, GERD symptoms will have improved, and an antireflux procedure will be unnecessary [13].

Upper endoscopy with esophageal biopsies can be used to evaluate patients for alternative diagnoses that can mimic GERD such as eosinophilic or infectious esophagitis. Endoscopy is indicated for pediatric patients who do not respond to a trial of medical therapy or present with anemia, hematemesis, or hemoccult positive stool. It is important to note that visual findings of erosive esophagitis are much less common in infants and children than in adults with GERD, and the gross appearance of the esophagus may not correlate well with histological findings. Thus, when upper endoscopy is employed in the evaluation of an infant or child with suspected GERD, esophageal biopsies are recommended [2].

Gastroesophageal scintigraphy or the "milk scan" has been used historically to document reflux in children. This study involves ingestion of a radiolabeled meal (i.e., milk in infants) and serial images to evaluate for passage of the contents from the stomach or back into the esophagus. This study can sometimes demonstrate episodes of GER and delayed gastric emptying, but the standards for interpretation of gastroesophageal scintigraphy in infants and children are not well-established. Thus, this test is not recommended in routine evaluation for pediatric GERD [1, 2].

Surgical Therapy for Pediatric GERD

Surgical treatment is indicated in pediatric patients with chronic GERD who have failed lifestyle changes and medical therapy, or who have life-threatening complications associated with their GERD. What constitutes an adequate trial of conservative management varies greatly with the age of the patient, the presenting symptoms, and the complications of GERD. Pediatric guidelines for the management of GERD outline several algorithms based on clinical presentatons, but the criteria for failure are not well-defined. In general, recurrence of symptoms or documented reflux esophagitis after withdrawal of antireflux medications is considered treatment failure. In young children, weight loss or failure to gain weight despite treatment are concerning signs, and apparent life-threatening events clearly associated with

GERD are indications to consider surgical therapy. Pediatric GERD guidelines emphasize the need for a thorough diagnostic workup to exclude non-GERD etiologies and appropriate family education and counseling about the risks of surgery, including the likelihood of fundoplication failure and symptom recurrence [1, 2], as well as the risks, benefits, and feasibility of any potential treatment options, such as long-term antireflux medical therapy or jejunal feedings.

The 360° Nissen fundoplication is the most commonly performed antireflux procedure in children, followed by the partial posterior Toupe fundoplication and anterior Thal fundoplication [15, 16]. Multiple studies have demonstrated the equivalent safety and efficacy of the laparoscopic vs. open approaches to fundoplication in pediatric patients, even in neonates and children with a history of laparotomy. Laparoscopic compared with open fundoplication results in a more rapid return to enteral feedings, shorter hospital stays, and decreased narcotic requirements in infants and children [16–20].

Several modifications to the standard surgical technique for fundoplication are recommended for pediatric patients. In infants, most fundoplications can be performed using 3 or 5 mm instruments through similar-sized ports or stab incisions. Insufflation pressures should be limited to 12 mmHg in infants, and a fundoplication length of 1.5–2.0 cm is suggested for patients weighing less than 3 kg. Bougie sizes for esophageal calibration are adjusted by weight, ranging from 20–24 French for 2.5–4.0 kg infants to 36–40 French for 10–15 kg young children. An 18 French nasogastric tube can be employed for very small premature infants [21].

One significant difference in the recommended fundoplication technique between adults and children involves the approach to dissection of the esophagus. In adults, extensive mobilization of the esophagus to create adequate intra-abdominal length is thought to be a critical part of the procedure [22, 23]. In children, growing evidence suggests that extensive esophageal dissection is not necessary and may in fact contribute to fundoplication failure by promoting transmigration of the wrap through the esophageal hiatus. Dissection of the esophagus at the hiatus was identified as a risk factor for re-do fundoplication in children, along with a younger age at first fundoplication and retching [24]. A single surgeon retrospective historical comparison demonstrated a decrease in the rate of wrap transmigration from 12 to 5 % by altering the surgical technique to perform minimal esophageal dissection, leaving the phrenoesophageal membrane intact and using two to four sutures to approximate the esophagus and the crura [25]. Further reductions were seen with time in this study as the number of esophagocrural sutures were increased from two to four. A two center, six surgeon, randomized controlled trial comparing maximal vs. minimal esophageal dissection demonstrated a decreased rate of wrap transmigration (30 % maximal vs. 7.8 % minimal) and a reduction in the rate of reoperation (18.4 % maximal vs. 3.3 % minimal) with minimal esophageal dissection [26]. All patients in this study underwent posterior crural approximation and placement of four esophagocrural sutures. With postoperative upper gastrointestinal contrast study at 1-year follow-up, this study demonstrated a significantly higher rate of wrap transmigration than previously reported. At 5-year follow-up, rates of wrap transmigration were 36.5 % for maximal dissection and 12.2 % for minimal dissection [27]. Thus, in pediatric patients, minimal dissection of the esophagus with preservation of the phrenoesophageal member is recommended to prevent wrap transmigration and reoperation. The role of esophagocrural sutures is controversial and currently the subject of a randomized controlled trial [28].

The efficacy of pediatric antireflux surgery was examined in a systematic review of prospective studies of antireflux operations in children [16]. Defining success as complete relief of symptoms, the median short-term success rate was 86 % (range 57–100 %) and the median long-term (i.e., >6 months) success rate was 72 % (range 70–96 %). Studies done in neurologically impaired children showed a lower median success rate of 70 % (range 57–79 %), but studies comparing neurologically impaired with normal children had variable results. Complication rates were highly variable, ranging from 0 to 54 %, with an increased rate seen in studies of neurologically impaired children. Dysphagia occurred in up to 33 % of patients, but was usually short-lived [16]. This review was limited in that failure was not well-defined in most studies, and complications were not well-reported.

Similar recurrence rates have been observed across surgical techniques including partial, total, open, and laparoscopic fundoplications in pediatric patients. Shorter hospital stays and decreased requirements for pain medications are seen with minimally invasive approaches [16]. Dysphagia is less common for partial vs. complete fundoplication [29]. In a randomized trial comparing Nissen and Thal fundoplications in children, there were no differences in short-term outcomes at 6 weeks after surgery, although dysphagia was more severe in children who underwent a Nissen fundoplication [30]. Long-term follow-up (i.e., median 30 months) revealed an absolute failure (i.e., recurrence requiring revision) rate that was significantly lower for Nissen (5.9 %) vs. Thal (15.9 %) fundoplications, with most failures occurring in neurologically impaired patients. There was not a significant difference in the rates of controlled recurrence of symptoms for Nissen (12.9 %) vs. Thal (9.8 %) fundoplications. The rates of dysphagia were similar for Nissen (23.5 %) and Thal (21.9 %) procedures, but the rates of severe dysphagia requiring endoscopy significantly were significantly greater in Nissen (24.7 %) vs. Thal (12.2 %) fundoplications [31].

Conclusions

In summary, GER is common in infants and children and must be carefully distinguished from GERD, which produces severe symptoms or complications. The gold standard test for the diagnosis of GERD in children is combined intraluminal esophageal pH monitoring and MII monitoring. Surgical treatment is indicated for patients with chronic GERD that is refractory to medical therapy or results in life-threatening complications. Parents should be carefully counseled about the risks and benefits of surgery, especially the rates of fundoplication failure. Minimal dissection of the esophagus at the hiatus with preservation of the phrenoesophageal membrane is recommended to prevent wrap transmigration. Complete Nissen fundoplication compared with partial fundoplication results in a lower failure rate, but higher likelihood of dysphagia requiring intervention.

References

1. Vandenplas Y, Rudolph CD, Di Lorenzo C, Hassall E, Liptak G, Mazur L, et al. Pediatric gastroesophageal reflux clinical practice guidelines: joint recommendations of the North American Society for Pediatric Gastroenterology, Hepatology, and Nutrition (NASPGHAN) and the European Society for Pediatric Gastroenterology, Hepatology, and Nutrition (ESPGHAN). J Pediatr Gastroenterol Nutr. 2009;49(4):498–547.
2. Lightdale JR, Gremse DA. Gastroesophageal reflux: management guidance for the pediatrician. Pediatrics. 2013;131(5):e1684–95.
3. Beyer JE, McGrath PJ, Berde CB. Discordance between self-report and behavioral pain measures in children aged 3-7 years after surgery. J Pain Symptom Manage. 1990;5(6):350–6.
4. Stanford EA, Chambers CT, Craig KD. A normative analysis of the development of pain-related vocabulary in children. Pain. 2005;114(1–2):278–84.
5. Stanford EA, Chambers CT, Craig KD. The role of developmental factors in predicting young children's use of a self-report scale for pain. Pain. 2006;120(1–2):16–23.
6. von Baeyer CL, Spagrud LJ. Systematic review of observational (behavioral) measures of pain for children and adolescents aged 3 to 18 years. Pain. 2007;127(1–2):140–50.
7. Francavilla R, Magista AM, Bucci N, Villirillo A, Boscarelli G, Mappa L, et al. Comparison of esophageal pH and multichannel intraluminal impedance testing in pediatric patients with suspected gastroesophageal reflux. J Pediatr Gastroenterol Nutr. 2010;50(2):154–60.
8. Mousa HM, Rosen R, Woodley FW, Orsi M, Armas D, Faure C, et al. Esophageal impedance monitoring for gastroesophageal reflux. J Pediatr Gastroenterol Nutr. 2011;52(2):129–39.
9. Rosen R, Hart K, Nurko S. Does reflux monitoring with multichannel intraluminal impedance change clinical decision making? J Pediatr Gastroenterol Nutr. 2011;52(4):404–7.
10. Aspelund G, Langer JC. Current management of hypertrophic pyloric stenosis. Semin Pediatr Surg. 2007;16(1):27–33.
11. Pandya S, Heiss K. Pyloric stenosis in pediatric surgery: an evidence-based review. Surg Clin North Am. 2012;92(3):527–39. vii–viii.
12. Valusek PA, St Peter SD, Keckler SJ, Laituri CA, Snyder CL, Ostlie DJ, et al. Does an upper gastrointestinal study change operative management for gastroesophageal reflux? J Pediatr Surg. 2010;45(6):1169–72.
13. Tiboni SG, Patel Y, Lander AD, Parikh DH, Jawaheer G, Arul GS. Management of gastroesophageal reflux associated with malrotation in children. J Pediatr Surg. 2011;46(2):289–91.
14. Lodwick DL, Minneci PC, Deans KJ. Current surgical management of intestinal rotational abnormalities. Curr Opin Pediatr. 2015;27(3):383–8.
15. Fonkalsrud EW, Ashcraft KW, Coran AG, Ellis DG, Grosfeld JL, Tunell WP, et al. Surgical treatment of gastroesophageal reflux in children: a combined hospital study of 7467 patients. Pediatrics. 1998;101(3):419–22.
16. Mauritz FA, van Herwaarden-Lindeboom MY, Stomp W, Zwaveling S, Fischer K, Houwen RH, et al. The effects and efficacy of antireflux surgery in children with gastroesophageal reflux disease: a systematic review. J Gastrointest Surg. 2011;15(10):1872–8.
17. Barsness KA, Feliz A, Potoka DA, Gaines BA, Upperman JS, Kane TD. Laparoscopic versus open Nissen fundoplication in infants after neonatal laparotomy. JSLS. 2007;11(4):461–5.
18. Kane TD. Laparoscopic Nissen fundoplication. Minerva Chir. 2009;64(2):147–57.
19. Pacilli M, Eaton S, McHoney M, Kiely EM, Drake DP, Curry JI, et al. Four year follow-up of a randomised controlled trial comparing open and laparoscopic Nissen fundoplication in children. Arch Dis Child. 2014;99(6):516–21.
20. Thatch KA, Yoo EY, Arthur 3rd LG, Finck C, Katz D, Moront M, et al. A comparison of laparoscopic and open Nissen fundoplication and gastrostomy placement in the neonatal intensive care unit population. J Pediatr Surg. 2010;45(2):346–9.
21. Ostlie DJ, Miller KA, Holcomb 3rd GW. Effective Nissen fundoplication length and bougie diameter size in young children undergoing laparoscopic Nissen fundoplication. J Pediatr Surg. 2002;37(12):1664–6.

22. Horgan S, Pellegrini CA. Surgical treatment of gastroesophageal reflux disease. Surg Clin North Am. 1997;77(5):1063–82.
23. Surgeons SSoAGaE. Guidelines for Surgical Treatment of Gastroesophageal Reflux Disease (GERD) 2010. http://www.sages.org/publications/guidelines/guidelines-for-surgical-treatment-of-gastroesophageal-reflux-disease-gerd/.
24. Baerg J, Thorpe D, Bultron G, Vannix R, Knott EM, Gasior AC, et al. A multicenter study of the incidence and factors associated with redo Nissen fundoplication in children. J Pediatr Surg. 2013;48(6):1306–11.
25. St Peter SD, Valusek PA, Calkins CM, Shew SB, Ostlie DJ, Holcomb 3rd GW. Use of esoph-agocrural sutures and minimal esophageal dissection reduces the incidence of postoperative transmigration of laparoscopic Nissen fundoplication wrap. J Pediatr Surg. 2007;42(1):25–9; discussion 9–30.
26. St Peter SD, Barnhart DC, Ostlie DJ, Tsao K, Leys CM, Sharp SW, et al. Minimal vs extensive esophageal mobilization during laparoscopic fundoplication: a prospective randomized trial. J Pediatr Surg. 2011;46(1):163–8.
27. Desai AA, Alemayehu H, Holcomb 3rd GW, St Peter SD. Minimal vs. maximal esophageal dissection and mobilization during laparoscopic fundoplication: long-term follow-up from a prospective, randomized trial. J Pediatr Surg. 2015;50(1):111–4.
28. ClinicalTrials.Gov. Prospective Randomized Trial Evaluating the Utility of Esophageal Stitches During Laparoscopic Fundoplication 2015. https://clinicaltrials.gov/ct2/show/NCT01509352. Accessed 5 July 2015
29. Weber TR. Toupet fundoplication for gastroesophageal reflux in childhood. Arch Surg. 1999;134(7):717–20; discussion 20–1.
30. Kubiak R, Andrews J, Grant HW. Laparoscopic Nissen fundoplication versus Thal fundoplication in children: comparison of short-term outcomes. J Laparoendosc Adv Surg Tech A. 2010;20(7):665–9.
31. Kubiak R, Andrews J, Grant HW. Long-term outcome of laparoscopic Nissen fundoplication compared with laparoscopic Thal fundoplication in children: a prospective, randomized study. Ann Surg. 2011;253(1):44–9.

Index

A
Anesthesia, 123
Anterior partial fundoplication
    achalasia, 109
    aorta lies posterior, 119
    crown sutures, 117, 118
    distal esophagus, 114
    dysphagia, 109
    esophageal hiatus, 114, 115, 119
    esophagus, 111, 114–116
    gastric fundus, 109
    gastro-esophageal junction, 109
    gastro-esophageal reflux disease, 110
    giant hiatus hernia, 118
    hiatal dissection and repair, 112–114
    hiatal repair suture, 116, 117
    high risk situations, 110
    and intra-abdominal position, 111
    left inferior phrenic artery, 119
    meta-analysis, 110
    outcomes, 119–120
    overweight and obese patients, 117
    positioning and port placement, 111–112
    postoperative care, 119
    randomized controlled trials, 110
    splenic hilum, 116
    stable flap valve, 117
    stomach, 116
    surgery, 110, 111, 119, 120
    vascular injury, 118
Antireflux surgery, 11, 13, 35, 71, 72

B
Barrett's esophagus, 133–135, 137

C
Collis gastroplasty
    dysphagia, 35
    fundoplication, 35
    gastroplasty, 35
    laparoscopic surgery, 34
    primary crural closure, 36
Computerized tomography (CT),
        26–27

D
Database, 130
Diaphragmatic crus
    component, 39
    drawback, 40
    esophageal hiatus, 39, 40
    falciform ligament, 40, 43–45
    gastropexy, 43, 51–52
    hiatal hernia, 39, 40
    hiatal tension, 40, 43
        esophageal hiatus, 46
        hiatal hernia, 46
        huntington's operative technique, 46
        intentional pneumothorax and
            diaphragmatic relaxing
            incisions, 45
    intentional pneumothorax, 40
    liver, 43
    primary hiatal closure, 42
    triangular ligament, 45
    types, mesh, 40
    unclosed hiatus, 42
    vascularized pedicle flaps, 43
Dysphagia, 35, 126, 127

© Springer International Publishing Switzerland 2016
R.W. Aye, J.G. Hunter (eds.), *Fundoplication Surgery*,
DOI 10.1007/978-3-319-25094-6

Printed in the United States
By Bookmasters